Manual of Urogynecology

AICOG 2018 Odisha

61st AICOG BHUBANESWAR 2018

Manual of
Urogynecology

Editors

SN Tripathy
KC Mahapatra
SK Giri
Vineet Mishra
Ajit Nayak

JAYPEE *The Health Sciences Publisher*
New Delhi | London | Panama

Jaypee Brothers Medical Publishers (P) Ltd

Headquarters

Jaypee Brothers Medical Publishers (P) Ltd
4838/24, Ansari Road, Daryaganj
New Delhi 110 002, India
Phone: +91-11-43574357
Fax: +91-11-43574314
Email: jaypee@jaypeebrothers.com

Overseas Offices

J.P. Medical Ltd
83 Victoria Street, London
SW1H 0HW (UK)
Phone: +44-20 317 08910
Fax: +44 (0)20 3008 6180
Email: info@jpmedpub.com

Jaypee-Highlights Medical Publishers Inc
City of Knowledge, Bld. 235, 2nd floor, Clayton
Panama City, Panama
Phone: +1 507-301-0496
Fax: +1 507-301-0499
Email: cservice@jphmedical.com

Jaypee Brothers Medical Publishers (P) Ltd
17/1-B Babar Road, Block-B, Shyamoli
Mohammadpur, Dhaka-1207
Bangladesh
Mobile: +08801912003485
Email: jaypeedhaka@gmail.com

Jaypee Brothers Medical Publishers (P) Ltd
Bhotahity, Kathmandu, Nepal
Phone: +977-9741283608
Email: Kathmandu@jaypeebrothers.com

Website: www.jaypeebrothers.com
Website: www.jaypeedigital.com

Inquiries for bulk sales may be solicited at: jaypee@jaypeebrothers.com

Manual of Urogynecology

First Edition: **2018**

ISBN 978-93-5270-372-2

Printed at: Samrat Offset Pvt. Ltd.

Contributors

A Tamilselvi
Consultant Urogynaecologist and Pelvic Floor Surgeon
Chennai, Tamil Nadu, India

Ajay Rane
Queensland, Australia

Anju Soni
Jaipur, Rajasthan, India

Jagdish Gandhi
East Yorkshire, England

Jay Iyer
Queensland, Australia

Narwadkar Mangesh
Nanded, Maharashtra, India

Rajamaheshwari
Chennai, Tamil Nadu, India

Subash Biswas
Kolkata, West Bengal, India

Suguna Kumar Veera
Vijayapur, Karnataka, India

Uma Rani Swain
Rohini, Delhi, India

Vineeth Mishra
Professor and Head
Department of Obstetric and Gynecology
Institute of Kidney Diseases and Research Center (IKDRC & ITS)
BJ Medical College
Ahmedabad, Gujrat, India

Message

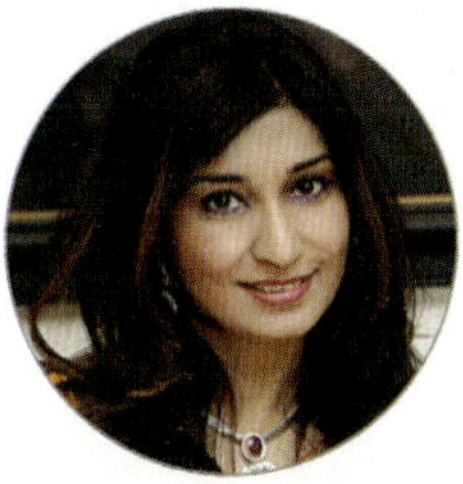

Rishma Dhillon Pai
MD DNB FCPS DGO FICOG
President, FOGSI—2017
Consultant Gynecologist
Jaslok Hospital, Lilavati Hospital and Hinduja Healthcare (Khar),
Bloom IVF Centre,
The Every Woman Clinic,
Mumbai, Maharashtra, India

"Wisdom.... comes not from age, but from education and learning."
Anton Chekhov

Life is a continuous process of learning. Especially in the field of medicine, which is constantly changing, it is very important to keep oneself abreast with the latest developments. It is heartening to note that academic workshop manuals are being released at the AICOG, Bhubaneswar, Odisha, India, for the benefit of the participating delegates and present varied updates in the field. Many different Manuals are being released on important subjects such as *3D Laparoscopy and Operative Oncology, Genetics, Fetal Medicine and Color Doppler, Postpartum Hemorrhage and High-Risk Pregnancy, Hysteroscopy,* etc.

I thank all the authors, for their immense contributions in building up the content for the manuals for Federation of Obstetric and Gynaecological Societies of India (FOGSI) by sharing their rich experiences in the field. These will be a big help to young gynecologists, who are still acquiring skills in various aspects of obstetrics and gynecology and a quick update for the seniors.

I extend congratulations to the organizing team of the AICOG 2018 and the editors of these manuals and wish you all success for this mega event.

"You cannot open a book without learning something."
—Confucius

Message

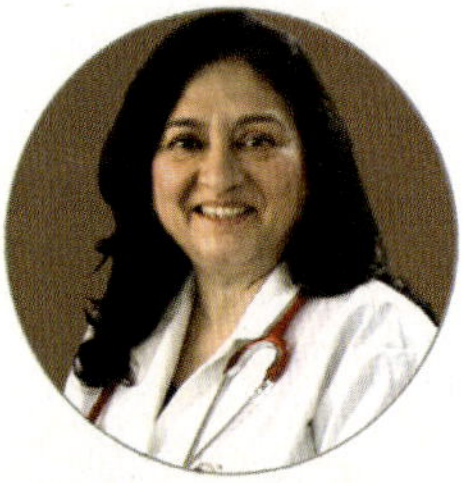

Jaideep Malhotra
MD FICMCH FICS FMAS FRCOG FICOG FRCPI FIAJAGO
Consultant ART (IVF)
President Elect, FOGSI—2018
Director, Rainbow IVF
Agra, Uttar Pradesh, India

"Education is greatest gift of life, it should never stop."

The subject of obstetrics and gynecology needs extreme proficiency as it deals with the medical specialties that focus on two different aspects. First one includes the care of pregnant women, the unborn baby, labor and delivery, as well as the immediate period following childbirth. Second aspect includes dealing with any ailment concerning the female reproductive organs. Hence, the manuals will help all those who are looking forward to gain excellence in the field of woman health. The manuals have tried to address all the issues a doctor needs.

With increasing expertise in all fields, the surgeon therefore while exercising a choice needs to follow the Hippocratic dictum—*"First, do no harm."*

We are thankful to all those who have incorporated their contribution by providing chapters from their research and collected scientific material and have shared their fruitful experiences for the delegates of the workshop.

As a part of my agenda for 2018, I as FOGSI President 2018, plan to work actively on QED (Quality, Ethics and Dignity) among our profession and also work towards HER (Health, Empowerment and Respect) towards our patients.

"Knowledge is of no value unless you put it into practices."

Message

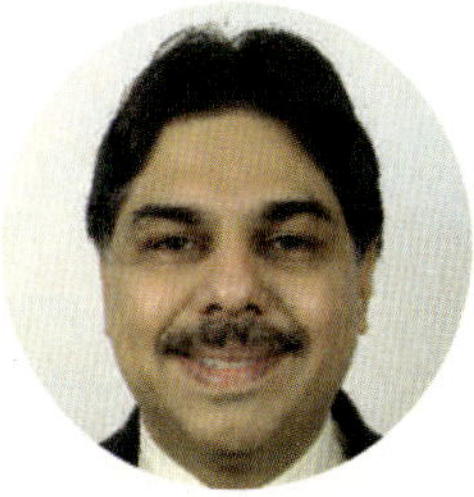

Hrishikesh Pai
Secretary General, FOGSI

It is my proud privilege to invite and welcome all delegates to the 61st All India Congress of Obstetrics and Gynaecology (AICOG) from 17th–21st January, 2018 at the Temple City of India, Bhubaneswar, Odisha, India.

It is propitious to note that the academic workshop manuals are being released which will reap beneficial reward to all the participating delegates.

I thank all the authors, for their immense contributions in building up the content for the manuals for Federation of Obstetric and Gynaecological Societies of India (FOGSI) by sharing their rich experiences in the field. These will be a big help to young gynecologists, who are still acquiring skills in various aspects of obstetrics and gynecology and a quick update for the seniors.

I forward my heartiest congratulations to all the contributors, the editors and the delegates of the workshop.

Message

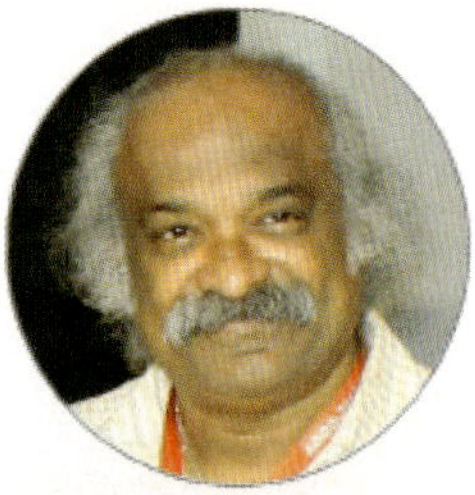

PC Mahapatra
Professor
Department of Obstetrics and Gynecology
SCB Medical College
Cuttack, Odisha, India
President, FOGSI—2011
Organising Chairperson

It is my proud privilege to invite and welcome all delegates to the 61st All India Congress of Obstetrics and Gynaecology (AICOG) from 17th–21st January, 2018 at the Temple City of India, Bhubaneswar, Odisha, India.

The five days of academic extravaganza will certainly enrich the scientific knowledge of all participating delegates and faculty. The precongress workshop on various aspects of this specialty will be held on 17th January 2018.

A quote by Edwin Louis Cole says that "*Winners are not those who never fail but those who never quit*" is apt for all the clinicians who are determined enough to see and overcome all the difficulties that are faced in the field of obstetrics and gynecology.

Today, with the advancement in the field of obstetrics and gynecology, everyone requires an in-depth knowledge of the complex subjects associated with the field so as to gain excellence in it.

This manual will prove to be a boon to all those who are associated with the field and wants to gain more knowledge in the subject matter.

Message

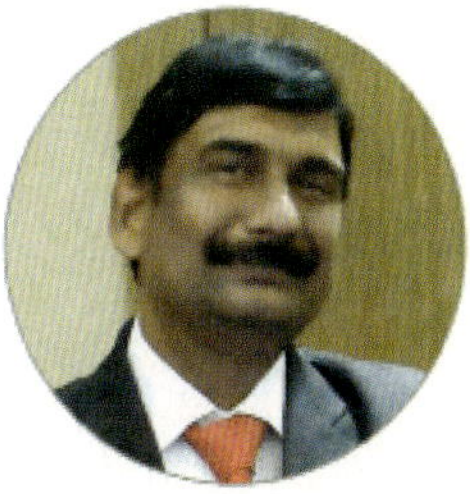

HP Pattanaik
Head
Department of Obstetrics and Gynecology
City Hospital
Cuttack, Odisha, India
Vice President, FOGSI—2009
Organising Secretary

Greetings from 61st AICOG 2018!
It is a matter of great pleasure to invite you all to 61st AICOG, from 17th–21st January, 2018 at the Temple City of India, Bhubaneswar, Odisha, India. The 11th Precongress workshops will be held on 17th January, 2018 in three medical colleges of Bhubaneswar.

It is propitious to note that the academic workshop manuals are being released which will reap beneficial reward to all the participating delegates.

It will also prove to be beneficial to the members of Federation of Obstetric and Gynaecological Societies of India (FOGSI), those who were unable to register themselves for the academic workshops.

I forward my heartiest congratulations to all the contributors, the editors and the delegates of the workshop.

Preface

"Man learns as he lives and experience is the greatest teacher in the world"
Swami Vivekananda

The act of micturition involve a very complex synergy between the higher centers, spinal reflexes and bladder whose prime aim is to store and void urine whenever the time is right. Urinary incontinence is involuntary leakage of urine and can happen as a disruption of any of the complex pathways or simply due to failure of bladder function. There are many types of incontinence.

Stress urinary incontinence is a major problem in younger women and older women have urge incontinence. A large number of women, especially older patients, are faced with a combination of stress and urge incontinence, the so-called mixed urinary incontinence. This is a very embarrassing condition. The woman hesitates to go out for fear of her leaking. If at all she goes out, she first searches for a washroom. Some studies have quoted a very high incidence in the elderly population. For treatment, it is very important to determine the type of incontinence, as the treatment for each types varies. There are many treatment options available at present apart from surgical management.

Vesicovaginal fistulas, as well as other urogenital fistulas, are very debilitating to patients. Early referral to individuals experienced in the management of fistula should be made, as the first repair attempt has the highest chance of closure via the vaginal route, the other routes of repair being abdominal, laparoscopy, etc.

Le Fort first described a new method for the cure of prolapsed uterus in 1877. The Le Fort partial colpocleisis is an obliterative vaginal procedure that approximates anterior and posterior vaginal walls. This surgery effectively replaces the prolapsed vaginal vaults into abdominal cavity with or without a uterus. It is indicated only in elderly women who have no future desire for sexual intercourse and having other concomitant medical disorders.

The noninvasive Vaginal Erbium: YAG SMOOTH laser (VEL) can be combined with the functional magnetic stimulation (FMS) for an efficacious and safe new method for the treatment of vaginal laxity, stress urinary incontinence, pelvic organ prolapses, vaginal atrophy. The VEL and FMS combine beautifully to treat tissue and muscle disorders and this type of combined therapy will soon become the treatment of choice for these indications.

Botulinum toxin (Botox) is a potent neurotoxin derived from Gram-positive anerobic spore-forming organism, *Clostridium Botulinum*. Type A (BOTOX) is currently used for the management of overactive bladder (OAB) symptoms caused by detrusor overactivity and for the patients who have not responded to the conservative management. Now there are several evidences to support its use for patient with OAB symptoms. The operative procedure is simple using a cystoscope. The beneficial effect lasts 6–9 months and a repeat injection may be necessary.

The principles involved in management of patients with UI, to achieve optimal results, include a broad understanding of the pathophysiology involved, a stepwise approach from conservative options like lifestyle modification, physiotherapy to more invasive therapies. Surgical skills has developed to a great extent and use of cystoscopy has reduced the risk of urinary tract injuries during pelvic surgery.

We hope that this workshop will help the delegates to understand the anatomy and physiology, evaluate the incontinence woman correctly and offer the latest therapy to the suffering humanity.

'He who learns and makes no use of the learning is a beast of burden with a load of books.'

Editors

Contents

Chapter 1

Surgical Anatomy of the Pelvic Floor

Dilgir S, Ajay Rane, Jay Iyer

DE LANCEY'S PELVIC FLOOR LEVELS (FIG. 1)

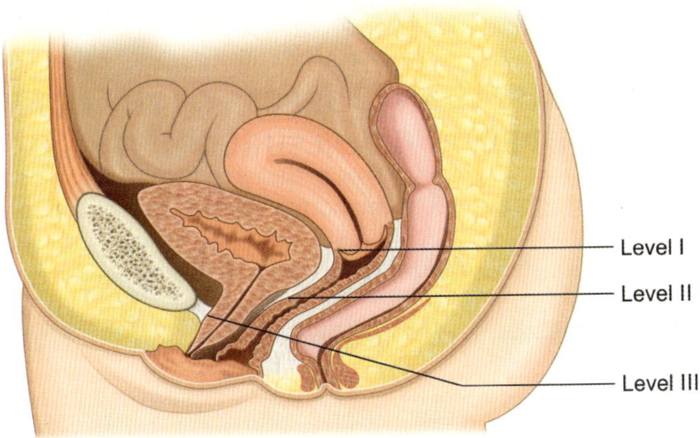

Fig. 1: Pelvic floor support levels.
Source: Porter et al. Pelvic floor support levels. 2008.

Table 1: Classification of pelvic floor levels.

Level	*Organs*	*Support*	*Pathology*	*Signs and symptoms*	*Treatment*
1 Apical	Uterus, cervix and vault	Uterosacral and cardinal ligaments	Utero (cervical), vault prolapse	Sensation of a bulge	Hysterectomy, hysteropexy
2 Anterior	Bladder	Fascial hammock	Cystocele	Sensation of a bulge, incomplete voiding and recurrent UTI	Anterior repair

Contd...

Contd...

Level	Organs	Support	Pathology	Signs and symptoms	Treatment
2 Posterior	Rectum	Fascial hammock	Rectocele	Sensation of a bulge and manual digitation	Posterior repair
3 Anterior	Urethra	Pubourethral ligament	Urethrocele	Urinary stress incontinence	Suburethral slings, bulking agents
3 Posterior	Perineal body	Perineal body, internal anal sphincter, and external anal sphincter	Enlarged genital hiatus	Sexual dysfunction and symptoms of vaginal laxity	Perineoplasty sphincter repairs

(UTI, Urinary tract infection).

SURGICALLY IMPORTANT ASPECTS OF THE BONY PELVIS TO THE PELVIC FLOOR SURGEON (FIG. 2)

Some of the important aspects of the bony pelvis to the pelvic floor surgeon are as follows:

- Sacral promontory: Useful landmark for surgical procedures of level 1 defects (e.g. sacrocolpopexy)
- Coccyx: Attachment for the levator ani muscles

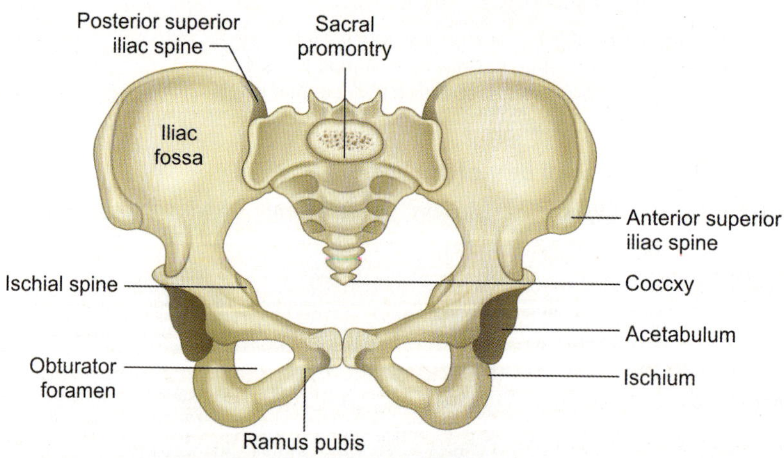

Fig. 2: Female bony pelvis.
Source: Sokol et al. Female bony pelvis (Gray's Anatomy of the Human Body, 1918). September. 2008.

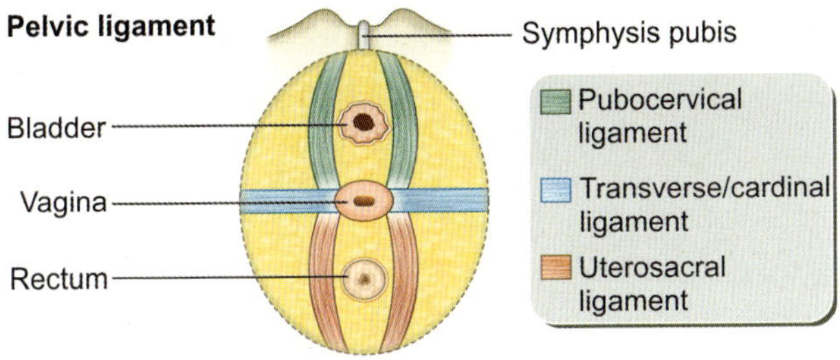

Fig. 3: Ligaments of the pelvic floor.
Source: Ker. Pelvic ligaments. Digital Image. 2012.

- Ischial spine: Landmark to perform pudendal block, identify the sacrospinous ligament (SSL)
- Anterior superior iliac spine (ASIS): Useful for port placement in laparoscopic surgery
- Pubic bone: Landmark for placement of transvaginal slings and the pectineal lines runs behind it.
- Obturator foramen: Import for placement of single incision slings and transobturator tapes.

LIGAMENTS OF THE PELVIC FLOOR OF IMPORTANCE TO THE PELVIC FLOOR SURGEON (FIG. 3)

- Uterosacral ligament: Level 1 support, composed of folds of peritoneum, attach to the cervix posterolaterally at the level of the internal cervical os. Anterior aspect of the ligaments attaches to the lateral vaginal fornices and posterior to the presacral fascia. Of great importance whist performing hysterectomies and providing level 1 support. Also, commonly involved in advanced endometriosis.
- Cardinal ligament: Level 1 support, attach to lateral aspect of cervix and upper third of vagina
- Pubocervical ligament: Ligament connecting the cervix to the posterior aspect of the symphysis pubis.

THE RELEVANCE OF THE PERINEAL MEMBRANE (UROGENITAL DIAPHRAGM) AND URETHRAL SUPPORT (FIG. 4)

- Perineal membrane: Consists of a sheet of dense connective tissue. Spans from the ischiopubic rami to the perineal body. The perineal membrane supports the urethra and vagina which pass through it
- Pubourethral ligaments: Not true ligaments as they are able to contract. They consist of an anterior, intermediate, and posterior component. Anterior aspect help stabilize urethra when there is a rise in intra-abdominal pressure.

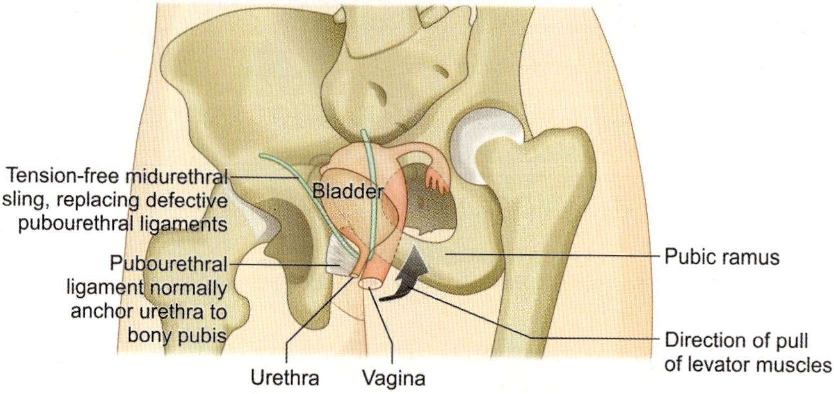

Fig. 4: Relevance of the perineal membrane (urogenital diaphragm) and urethral support. *Source:* Smit et al. Digital Image. Action of tension-free midurethral sling in treatment of stress urinary incontinence in women. 2006.

Damage to these, results in urethral hypermobility and defective anchoring. Suburethral slings act to mimic these ligaments

- Intrinsic urethral sphincter: Composed of smooth muscles under autonomic control.
- Striate urogenital sphincter: Composed of three muscle groups and are under voluntary control and also provide one-third of the resting tone. Innervated by branches of the pudendal nerve.

THE PELVIC DIAPHRAGM AND ITS IMPORTANCE TO THE PELVIC FLOOR SURGEON

- Pelvic diaphragm is composed of levator ani muscles and inferior and superior fascia (Fig. 5)
- Pubococcygeus: Main component of the levator ani muscles which inserts to the pubic bone at a distance 1.5 cm from the symphysis to insert to the levator plate
- Iliococcygeus: Originates from the obturator internus fascia, runs along the arcus tendineus levator ani muscle inserts to the lateral margin of the coccyx and lower sacrum
- Puborectalis: U-shaped muscle which extends from pubic bone, past urogenital hiatus creating a 90° 'sling' around the anorectal junction. Sits in a tonic contracted state.
- Coccygeus: Not part of levator ani complex however, forms posterior part of the pelvic floor. Spans from ischial spine and inserts on the lateral margin of the coccyx and lower sacrum. It is located on the superior aspect of the SSL.

Birth trauma is a major risk factor for trauma to the levator ani complex. This can be identified clinically by palpating for the insertion of the muscles beneath inferior pubic ramus. Alternatively, it can be identified using three-dimensional/four-dimensional (3D/4D) translabial ultrasound (Fig. 6).

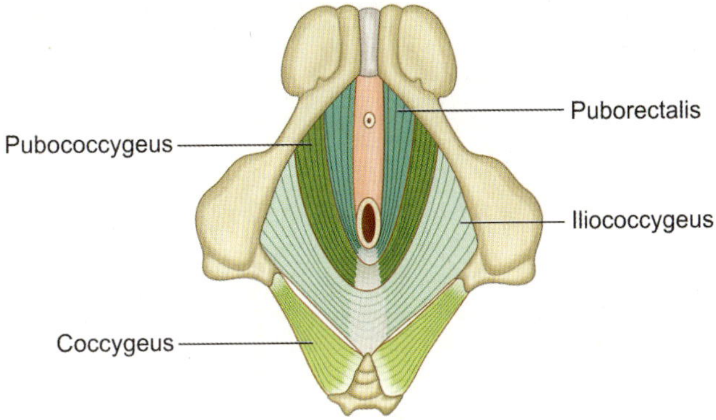

Fig. 5: Levator ani muscles.
Source: Teach Me Anatomy. Digital Image. 2017.

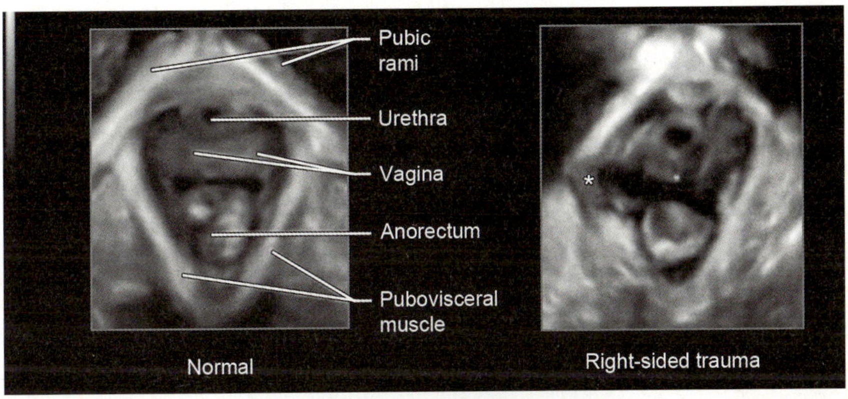

Fig. 6: Birth trauma.
Source: Dietz. Digital Image. Sydney. 2014.

EPISIOTOMY (FIG. 7)

Structures that are cut during a mediolateral episiotomy include: vaginal epithelium, perineal muscle, bulbocavernosus muscle and perineal skin. Often health care professionals are unaware of the exact angle to perform an episiotomy especially given the that the perineum is at a stretch during crowning. This can lead to obstetric anal sphincter injury (OASI) as the angle is often too medial. Therefore, we are conducting a trial on a tool known as an episiometer which would facilitate an episiotomy to be made at approximately a 60° angle, thereby minimizing OASI.

The episiometer (Fig. 8) is a tool used in our hospital that is placed on the laboring women's perineum when performing an episiotomy. This facilitates formation of an episiotomy at approximately a 60° angle, thereby minimizing obstetric anal sphincter injury.

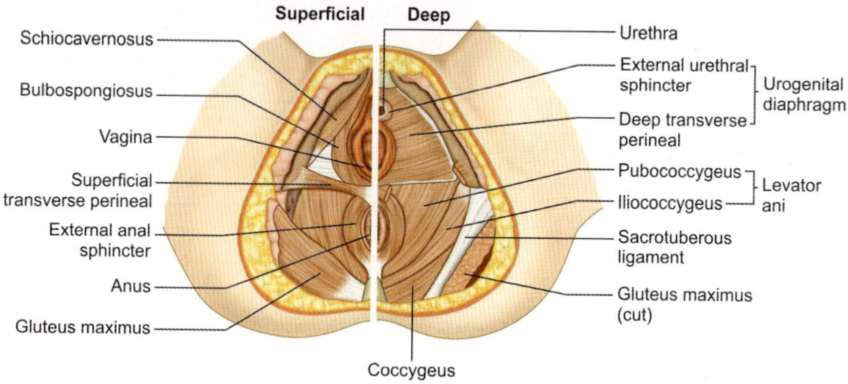

Fig. 7: Episiotomy.
Source: Thepregnantpt. Digital Image. 2014.

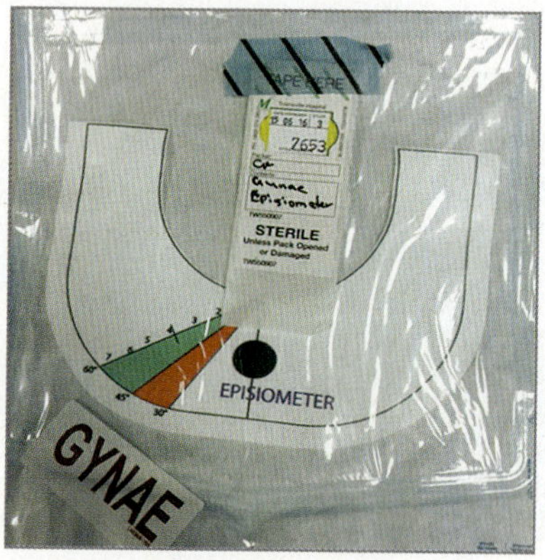

Fig. 8: Episiometer.

BLOOD SUPPLY TO PELVIC FLOOR OF IMPORTANCE TO THE PELVIC FLOOR SURGEON (FIG. 9)

ARTERIES OF THE FEMALE PERINEUM (FIG. 10)

Internal iliac artery is the major artery that supplies the pelvic structures. At the greater sciatic foramen, it further subdivides into the anterior and posterior trunks. Details of the subdivision will not be discussed. However, it is important to realize that level 3 structures receive the most dense blood supply from the pudendal arteries. Therefore, during vaginal surgery the surgeon may note that operating in the level 3 results in most blood loss.

Inferior rectal artery and vein are exposed during dissection to identify the transverse perineal muscles while performing a perineoplasty. The muscles are united during this procedure.

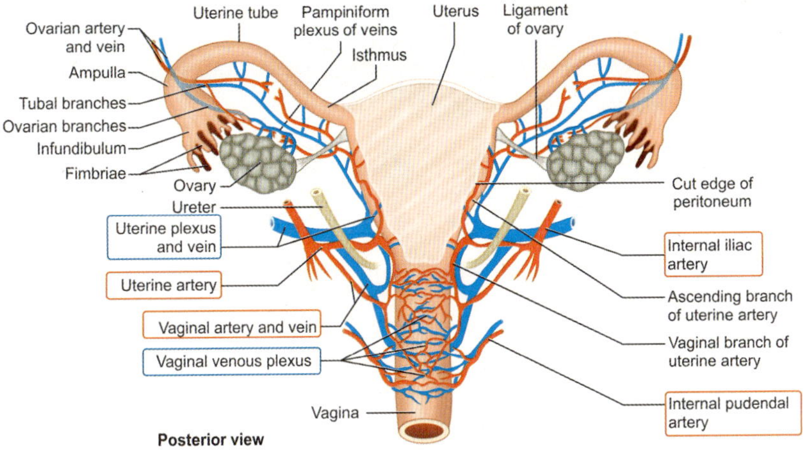

Fig. 9: Posterior view of anatomy of female reproductive organs the blood supply to pelvic floor.
Source: Daha. Digital Image. Anatomy of female reproductive organs. 2017.

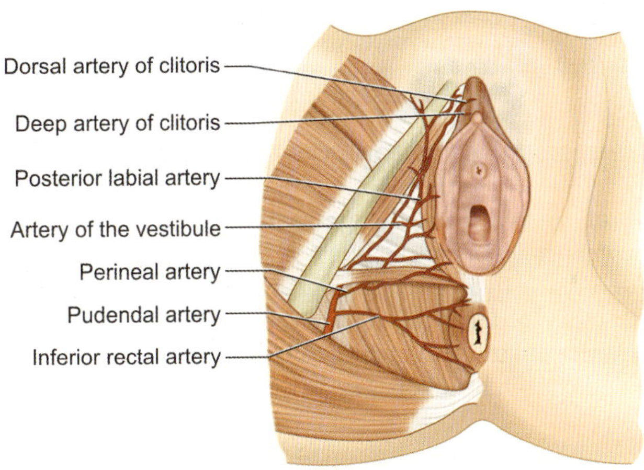

Fig. 10: Surgical female urogenital anatomy showing arteries of the female perineum.
Source: UpToDate. Digital Image. Surgical Female Urogenital Anatomy. 2017.

POTENTIAL STRUCTURES SUSCEPTIBLE TO DAMAGE DURING ACCESS TO SACROSPINOUS LIGAMENT (FIG. 11)

Pudendal block is a commonly performed procedure. Local anesthetic is injected 1 cm posterior and medial to the ischial spine. SSL fixation involves placing a stitch to SSL in order to provide level 1 support. The pudendal vein, artery, and nerve are at risk during these commonly performed procedures. Branches of the sciatic nerve can also get injured by the SSL suture. Buttock pain is a known risk, secondary to nerve entrapment and may even require release of the sacrospinous stitch.

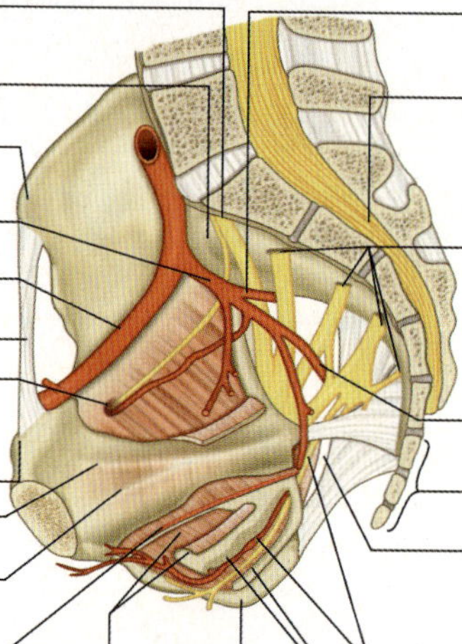

Fig. 11: Sacrospinous ligament complex.
Source: Access Medicine. Digital Image. Sacrospinous ligament complex adapted from Williams Gynaecology ed2.

URETERIC INJURY AT TIME OF VAGINAL SURGERY

Risk of ureteral injury during a vaginal hysterectomy is anywhere from 0.1–0.5%. Ureter is mostly at risk of injury during a vaginal hysterectomy at the level of the uterosacral ligaments, uterine vessels and when the angles of the vagina are closed. In order to avoid injury, it is import to reflect the bladder and provide downward traction to the cervix in a down and opposite direction to where the pedicle will be taken (Fig. 12).

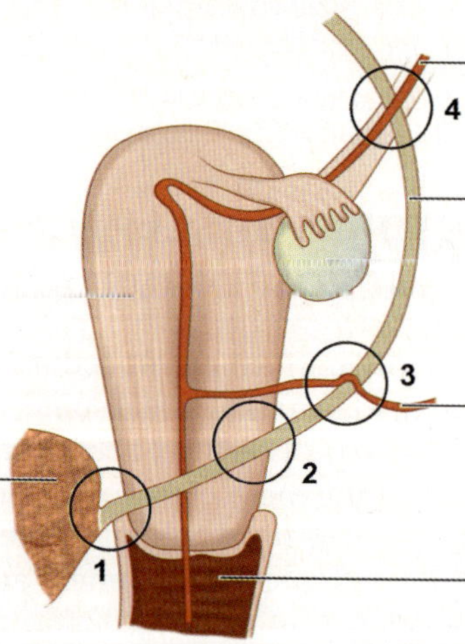

Fig. 12: Major ureter reconstruction.
Source: Major Ureter Reconstruction. Digital Image. 2016.

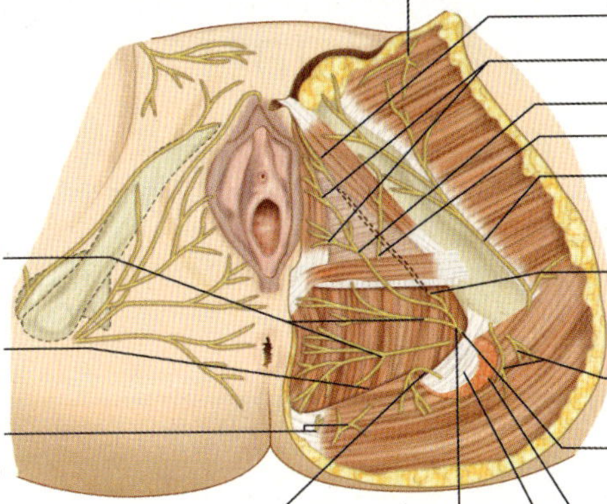

Fig. 13: Nerve supply to pelvic floor.
Source: Kurkakula. Digital Image. Pelvic Floor. 2015.

NERVE SUPPLY TO THE PELVIC FLOOR

Injury to the pelvic floor nerves is not uncommon during childbirth and secondary to surgery. This can result in reduced sensation or incontinence. Furthermore, awareness of the nerve supply to the pelvic floor is of utmost importance when conducting assessment for chronic pelvic pain, vaginismus or vulvodynia. Pudendal neuralgia is a condition that can often present with pain in the clitoris, labia, vagina, urethra, perineum, anus or rectum. Understanding the distribution of the pudendal nerve allows one to have a better understanding of the cause of the pathology (Fig. 13).

Chapter 2

Clinical Evaluation of Pelvic Organ Prolapse

N Rajamaheswari

Pelvic organ prolapse (POP) is a frequently encountered problem which compromises quality of life of women. Ensuring successful outcome with no future recurrence or complications is unquestionably a challenge. Emergence of newer concepts on supports of pelvic organs and better understanding of the anatomy of the pelvic floor has enhanced our knowledge.

Meticulous evaluation leads to an accurate diagnosis which is essential to plan appropriate management. Clinical evaluation defines the degree of prolapse objectively and ensures subjective assessment of integrity of connective tissue and muscular support of pelvic organs. Evaluation may be performed in sitting or standing position. Examination in dorsal lithotomy is simpler and preferred by clinicians even though it may mask the severity of prolapse. Evaluation is done by way of inspection and palpation with the help of simple instruments like speculum and retractors at rest and straining position. Digital examination includes vaginal, bimanual, rectal, and rectovaginal examination.

Bimanual examination identifies tenderness, location, size, mobility of uterus, cervix, bladder, and adnexa. Recognizing coexisting mass is crucial. Bimanual and rectovaginal examination enables assessment of connective tissue and muscular support of pelvic organs. Evaluation starts with anterior vagina followed by posterior vagina and apex and assessment of support at all levels should be performed.

Examination of anterior vagina with the speculum facilitates assessing urethra, urethrovaginal junction, and bladder. Inspection of vagina, cervix, uterus, and perineum is necessary. Assessment of descent and its extent, vaginal epithelium (color effect of estrogen), vaginal rugosity, obliteration of sulci, and perineal concavity should be done in order. Pink and supple vagina indicates well-estrogenized status and presence of rugosity certifies intact underlying visceral connective tissue. A persistent bulge in anterior vaginal wall (with support) but without rugosity suggest a central defect in pubocervical fascia. However, a bulge with rugosity with loss of anterolateral sulci suggests a paravaginal defect. Such bulge disappears if support provided to the lateral fornices by an instrument (support test).

Transverse tear of pubocervical fascia from anterior margin of pericervical ring results in bulge in anterior fornix (without rugosity). Transverse separation of pericervical ring from uterosacral ligament with intact pubocervical fascia causes descent of cervix/vault. Examination of posterior vaginal wall may reveal transverse rugosity or bulging rectum against vaginal epithelium when the support is defective.

Separation of rectovaginal fascia from uterosacral ligament results in bulge in posterior fornix. Intact uterosacral ligament with separation of fascia may result in elongation of cervix. A rectovaginal examination may differentiate a low from high rectocele. Enterocele is diagnosed by rectovaginal examination if a loop of bowel felt. Anterior and posterior wall descent mostly coexists. Apical defect manifesting as uterine descent or as vault prolapse are not difficult to diagnose. Assessing the side-to-side and vertical mobility of the prolapse should be done. Separation of cervix from cardinal ligaments causes wide lateral mobility of cervix. Separation of cervix from uterosacral ligament causes vertical mobility.

It is essential to identify associated decubitus ulcer, premalignant, or malignant lesions over the vaginal wall. Irreducibility of prolapse secondary to uterine tumor, big bladder stone, or impacted mass in polycystic ovarian disease (POD) should be recognized. Examination of perineum by inspection and palpation is vital. Presence of perineal concavity is normal.

Visualizing and palpating the pelvic floor during a voluntary contraction recognizing muscle body insertion, its strength, duration of contraction, and anterior lift during contraction are essential. Normal location of perineum is at ischial tuberosities or within 2 cm below it. Location of perineum beyond 2 cm at rest or straining is referred perineal descent. Vaginal, rectal-and rectovaginal examination should identify the integrity of rectovaginal septum, enterocele, and laxity of anal sphincter.

Describing and comparing POP to a known volume is imprecise and inconsistent. Hence, pelvic organ prolapse quantification (POP-Q), a universally accepted system, is adopted to describe the anatomic position of pelvic organs. Hymen is used as reference point and nine measurements made to plot the POP-Q grid. POP-Q quantifies and aids in understanding POP. It describes the degree of compromise of supporting tissue; however, it does not identify the underlying defect.

It is essential to diagnose and address coexisting uterine tumor, bladder stone, cystic and solid mass in the vagina, rectal prolapse, urethral mucosal prolapse, and sphincter incompetence in order to obtain successful outcome. Imaging modalities like X-rays, computed tomography (CT), and magnetic resonance imaging (MRI) are rarely required though ultrasound imaging is frequently used as an adjunct. Transperineal imaging is valuable in diagnosing enterocele. Clinicians need to be aware of mixed defects in different levels in order to plan the appropriate management and to optimize the success. Identifying coexisting dysfunctions and addressing the pelvic floor as a complete entity will enable us to achieve the goals of reconstructive pelvic floor surgery. Adopting the POP-Q will enable objective assessment of outcome after surgery.

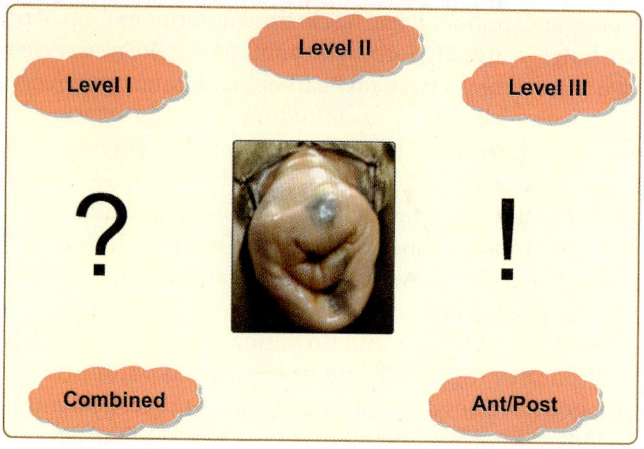

Fig. 1

BIBLIOGRAPHY

1. Brubaker L, Glazener C, Jacquetin B, et al. Surgery for Pelvic Organ Prolapse: Incontinence. 4th edition. 4th International Consultation on Incontinence: Health publications limited; 2009. pp. 1275-310.
2. Haessler AL, Lin LL, Ho MH, et al. Reevaluating occult incontinence. Curr Opin Obstet Gynecol. 2005;17(5):535-40.
3. Maher C, Baessler K, Glazener CM, et al. Surgical management of pelvic organ prolapse in women. Cochrane Database Syst Rev. 2007;(3):CD004014.
4. Maher C, Feiner B, Baessler K, et al. Surgical management of pelvic organ prolapse in women. Cochrane Database Syst Rev. 2004;(4):CD004014.
5. Shull BL, Capen CV, Riggs MW, et al. Preoperative and postoperative analysis of site-specific pelvic support defects in 81 women treated with sacrospinous ligament suspension and pelvic reconstruction. AM J Obstet Gynecol. 1992;166(6 Pt 1):1764-8.
6. Wertz RW, Wertz DC. Lying-in: A history of childbirth in America. New Haven, CT: Yale University Press; 1989.

Chapter 3

Surgical Procedures for Pelvic Organ Prolapse

Uma Rani Swain

Pelvic organ prolapse (POP) is an entity of multifactorial origin, and to name a few, congenital weakness of connective tissue, trivial injuries to pelvis floor during vaginal deliveries, age-related laxity and weakness in menopause believed to be the main causative factors.

Vaginal child births cause detachment, denudation and denervation of pelvic floor supports especially during difficult deliveries like big baby, prolonged 2nd stage of labor, instrumental deliveries as a result of which pelvic floor loses its tone and strength. Increase intra-abdominal pressure exaggerates its ballooning effects and hypoestrogenic state of menopause accelerates the severity and prolapse sets in.

Depending on the site of defects, De Lancey classifies pelvic organ prolapse (POP) as Level I (vault/apex of vagina), II (mid vagina), III (distal vagina and introitus).

Pelvic reconstructive surgery remains the mainstay of treatment and vaginal route is commonly preferred.

PRINCIPLE OF SURGERY

Level I Defects

Patient presents with a perineal bulge consists of uterocervical descent along with a part or the whole length of vagina. The defect lies at the apex of vagina and pericervical ring (pubocervicovaginal fascia, rectovaginal fascia and uterosacral—cardinal ligament complex).

Uterosacral ligament (USL) is considered to be the main support at vaginal cuff and cervix. Suspension procedures are proved to be highly effective and thus recommended for Level I defects.

PRINCIPLE

We select a point in any ligament of pelvis which is strong enough to hold the prolapsed organ in place and also can sustain the intra-abdominal and pelvis pressure constantly. Not only this should reduce the bulge but also maintain the bladder, bowel and sexual functions.

According to the ligaments selected for suspension of the vault, different surgical procedures are named accordingly.

High Uterosacral Ligament Suspension

Here the intermediate part of uterosacral ligament is selected for this purpose. This portion of USL is easy to identify, strong enough and maintains reasonable distance from ureter.

Bilateral suspension is commonly performed to maintain the anatomical axis, length and symmetry of vagina. USL can be approached intra- or extra-peritoneal depending on the expertise of the surgeon.

It is a very effective, durable and patient friendly procedure if done properly. Ureteric complication (kinking, injury, obstruction due to ligature) is 1% to 13%. So, postoperative cystoscopy is advocated to confirm ureteric patency.

Sacrospinous Ligament Suspension (Unilaterally/bilaterally)

Here the suspension point is medial part of sacrospinous ligament (SSL). This procedure can be done unilaterally or bilaterally according to the length and width of vagina available for a tension free-suspension. There are different types of needles or ligature carriers available to ease out the suturing through the ligament because the depth of pararectal space over this ligament is very limited.

The procedure is extraperitoneal, the complications related to laparotomy are rare but care should be taken to avoid handling the lateral portion of SSL which can lead to injury to structures like lateral sacral nerve, pudendal neurovascular bundles and posterior gluteal vessel.

McCall's Culdoplasty

It is more suitable in case of enterocele as Level I defect where distal part of USL is selected to reduce the enterocele.

Internal McCall's sutures are taken by nonabsorbable sutures to bring both USL to midline and obliterate the cul-de-sac whereas external McCall's suture suspends the posterior lip of vaginal cuff with delayed absorbable sutures.

The number of internal sutures depends on the severity of enterocele.

As this procedure involves USL, postoperative cystoscopy is advisable to avoid ureteric complications. Rectal injury and rectovaginal fistula are reported as complications so thorough rectal examination should be done for diagnosis.

Abdominal Sacrocolpopexy/Hysteropexy

Here anterior longitudinal ligament over sacrum is selected as suspension point and a long piece of nonabsorbable mesh is used to suspend the vault to sacrum. It maintains vaginal length and axis near to its anatomy.

This procedure can be done by laparotomy/laparoscopy/Robotic and it carries all risks of open surgery.

Modified Khanna's Sling

It is recommended in younger patients where preservation of uterus is desired, i.e. hysteropexy. Here the midpoint of a long strip of nonabsorbable mesh is attached to the posterior aspect of cervix through colpotomy and through laparoscope retroperitoneally a tunnel is created over the lateral wall of pelvis. Through this tunnel one end of mesh strip is retrieved and fixed to the ligament medial to anterior superior iliac spine. The same is repeated on the other side to achieve a desired level of suspension of uterus.

Prolapse in Short Vagina

Best suited for sacrocolpopexy or any obliterative procedures (colpocleisis).

Level II Defects

Include cystocele (anterior), rectocele (posterior) and lateral protrusions of vaginal wall. They can be presented alone or along with Level I defects.

Mid vagina is supported by pubocervical vaginal fascia anteriorly and rectovaginal fascia posteriorly which get attached to arcus tendineus fascia pelvis (ATFP) on an either side forming lateral fornix. So, the reconstructive procedures aim to correct those defects through site specific repair, vaginal paravaginal defect repairs, midline placation of endopelvic fascia (anterior and posterior colporrhaphy).

Level III Defects

It is the defect of distal part of vagina present in form of urethrocele anteriorly and perineocele posteriorly.

Urethrocele can be repaired with midline plication of pubourethral ligament.

As the perineal body represents the conglomeration of several superficial perineal muscles and fascia, perineoceal repair includes midline fusion of these structures giving rise to thick and lengthy perineal body.

Selection criteria of different procedures depend mostly on the skill and expertise of surgeon. Preoperative vaginal length should be good enough to allow the proximal vagina getting attached to the suspension point without any suture bridge or tension thus gives rise to robust support to vaginal apex in future.

Preoperative counseling of patient must include the type of surgery selected, associated complications and percentage of success in relieving the symptoms. Ultimately all reconstructive procedures should address the patient symptoms simultaneously maintaining the physiology of bladder and bowel with special attention to sexual function.

Chapter 4

Surgical Management of Vesicovaginal Fistula

Mangesh Narwadkar

INTRODUCTION

Vesicovaginal fistulas (VVF), as well as other urogenital fistulas, are very debilitating to patients. Early referral to individuals experienced in the management of fistula should be made, as the first repair attempt has the highest chance of closure via the vaginal route. Successful repair can be expected in 80–90% of patients, but multiple surgeries may be required. These patients should be evaluated when they first become symptomatic and by practitioners experienced in treating these conditions.

Surgical treatment of benign pelvic condition causes approximately 90% VVF with total abdominal hysterectomy being the most common cause.

Many fistulas occur secondary to trauma, crushing injuries from clamps, or suture penetration into the lower urinary tract, which may result in devascularization, necrosis and invariably fistulous development between the second and tenth postoperative day.

The best management of urogenital fistulae, other than prevention, is the recognition and repair of the injury at the primary surgery. If VVF, is diagnosed within 7 days of occurrence, is less than 1 cm in diameter and unrelated to malignancy or radiation, continuous bladder drainage alone up to 4 weeks allows postoperative healing in 12–80% of cases, however the outcome is unpredictable.

EARLY REPAIR

The timing of fistula repair is dependent on the surgical-readiness of the surrounding tissue. If the tissue is healthy, early repair can be done. Otherwise 6–12 weeks are sufficient to allow most granulation tissue to dissipate, increasing the chance of a successful repair. During the waiting period, catheterization of the bladder may decrease symptoms and allow for spontaneous closure.

Most VVF can be closed transvaginally. Simple VVF are usually repaired with the Latzko technique, whereas more complex procedures usually require excision of the tract and a layered closure of the defect. If the fistula approaches on one or both ureteral orifices the ureters should be catheterized at the onset of surgery.

Intraoperative placement of the pediatric Foley catheter through the fistula and into the bladder helps to evert the fistula edge, thus improving descent and stability for dissection.

Latzko (Partial Colpocleisis)

The reported cure rates are in between 93% and 100% after the first attempt. This simple procedure offers advantage of short operating time, minimal blood loss and low postoperative morbidity.

In this, vaginal mucosa is mobilized around the fistula margin in the shape of ellipse for at least 2.5 cm in all direction.

Closure of subvaginal tissue and vaginal mucosa is done in layers using 2.0 or 3.0 interrupted absorbable sutures.

Complicated or Larger Fistula

- A classic technique is best
- Circumscribe the vaginal mucosa in the region of the fistula
- Sufficient vaginal mucosa is separated from the underlying pubocervical fascia to permit tension-free closure
- Traction on the scar tissue and countertraction on the edges of vaginal mucosa is to facilitate accurate undermining of the vagina
- Subvaginal plane is dissected in all directions
- If the fistulous tract is small completely excise it
- If tract is large and fibrotic, the edge should be freshened
- Avoid overexcision to avoid larger defect and postoperative bleeding from the bladder which causes catheter blockage, bladder distention and failure of the repair.
- Layered closure is performed
- The first layer involves interrupted 3-0 delayed absorbable in an extra-mucosal fashion, extending lateral to the fistulous opening. All sutures placed and then individually tied
- This suture line is inverted and second suture line of similar sutures is placed through the muscular portion of the wall of bladder. This suture row will imbricate the first one
- At this stage you can test the integrity of the repair by instilling methylene blue in the bladder. (but avoid overdistention)
- Third layer of suture in pubocervical fascia over the fistulous closure
- The vaginal epithelium is closed with delayed absorbable 2-0 sutures
- Vaginal packing for 24 hours
- Postoperative catheter for 2 weeks with transurethral Foley catheter.

ABDOMINAL REPAIR OF VESICOVAGINAL FISTULA

- *Indications:* High and inaccessible fistula, multiple fistula, involvement of uterus or bowel and the need for urethral reimplantation
- Midline or transverse skin incision
  - Midline—allows easier access to the abdomen for retrieval and mobilization of omentum
  - Transverse—use muscle splitting incision such as Maylard or Cherney incision
- Once the peritoneum has been opened, the bowel is packed posteriorly and usually a self-retaining retractor is placed. The bladder is then exposed and a high extraperitoneal intentional cystotomy is made
- The fistulous tract is then visualized from the inside of the bladder
- If it is in close proximity to the ureteral orifices, ureteral stents should be placed. They can be placed via a cystoscopic approach or intraoperatively via a transvesical approach
- The bladder incision is then taken down along the back of the bladder all the way to the fistulous tract
- The fistulous tract is completely excised, and the vagina is sharply mobilized off the back of the bladder
- A pack of EEA™ sizer placed in the vagina will produce vaginal distention and facilitates countertraction, which assists the dissection. Traction and countertraction on the vagina and bladder facilitate short accurate separation of these two surfaces
- It is important to proceed with this dissection well beyond any scarification produced by the fistula. The vagina is then closed with interrupted 2-0 absorbable sutures, preferably in two layers
- The bladder is closed with 3-0 absorbable sutures in a running fashion or with the interrupted sutures. The bladder is also preferably closed in two layers
- It is usually advantageous to mobilize a piece of omentum down to the site of the fistula repair. It is sutured to the anterior wall of the vagina or the posterior wall of the bladder to thus give additional blood supply and a tissue barrier between the suture lines
- Catheter drainage may be accomplished with a transurethral or suprapubic catheter (or both), depending on the extent and circumstances of the repair.

Chapter 5

Urinary Tract Injury in Urogynecological Surgery

Subhash Chandra Biswas

INTRODUCTION

The genital organs and urinary tract arise in the intermediate mesoderm on either side of the root of the mesentery beneath the epithelium of the coelom. Subsequent growth and development of the two systems make an intimate anatomic relationship between them. This close proximity, embryologically and anatomically, predisposes the lower urinary tract (UT) at risk of trauma during urogynecologic surgery. Approximately, in 1–2% of gynecological surgeries result in UT injuries. Up to 90% of lower UT injuries occur in gynecologic surgeries. Majority of those injuries, if not all, are avoidable. This article emphasizes on the prevention and principles of management of those injuries.

SURGICAL PROCEDURES ATTRIBUTABLE

The most common gynecological surgery accountable to such injury is hysterectomy, be it vaginal, abdominal, or laparoscopic approach. Other procedures attributable to UT trauma are surgery for pelvic organ prolapse (POP), myomectomy, oophorectomy, removal of tubo-ovarian mass, and adhesiolysis. Excision of vaginal cyst in anterolateral wall may traumatize bladder with urethra. Newer surgical procedures [transobturator (TOT); transvaginal obturator (TVT-O), TVT] for stress urinary incontinence (SUI) can cause bladder and urethral injuries. The risk is increased in radical surgery, pelvic inflammatory disease (PID) and endometriosis, and adhesions due to previous surgery.

Ureteric injuries are of varying degrees like partial or complete laceration, segmental excision, suture transfixation, kinking/angulation, ligature, crushing, and stripping/ischemic injuries and cautery/thermal injuries. Bladder and urethra are also liable to be traumatized in the similar way. This may result in fistulous communication between the two tracts.

Prevention of Injuries

Preoperative evaluation by taking detailed history, physical examination, and laboratory evaluation may identify the subjects at increased susceptibility during any procedure. Evaluation is essential by imaging (USG/MRI), endoscopy, and multidisciplinary consultation. Sonography may detect ureteral obstruction, stricture, and anatomical deviation and estimate residual urinary volume. Intravenous urogram (IVU) documents anatomic abnormalities, defines renal function, and localizes ureteric obstruction. It is important in evaluation of genitourinary fistula. Cystourethroscopy is indicated in preoperative evaluation of hematuria, abnormal urinary cytology, recurrent UTI, urinary fistula, urethral or bladder diverticula, subjects with incontinence, and staging of gynecological malignancies to define extent and nature of surgery. The urine should be tested for infection before surgery.

Intravenous urography is valuable in the evaluation of genitourinary fistulas; it documents anatomic abnormalities, defines renal function, and localizes ureteric obstruction. Retrograde pyelograms are helpful in locating ureteral obstructions and fistulas.

Preoperative retrograde ureteral stent or catheter placement has not been shown to reduce the incidence of surgical injury to the ureter. The procedure itself may cause bleeding, edema, and perforation of the ureter. The stent is often difficult to feel within an area of fibrosis, and it might impart immobility to the ureter, so predisposes the ureter to damage.

Intraoperative Care

Good lighting, positioning, adequate exposure, and maintenance of sterile techniques are essential and a transurethral catheter for emptying and filling the bladder are recommended. During all surgical procedures, sharp dissection is preferable to blunt dissection. Taking small pedicles is preferred to taking large pedicles. When hemostasis is a problem, pressure should be applied until the bleeding vessel can be identified and selectively clamped. Many ureters are damaged by the application of clamps in a frantic effort to control pelvic hemorrhage.

Abdominal Approach

Abdominal incisions should be made to allow adequate exposure of the entire pelvis. The peritoneal cavity is entered as high as possible to avoid direct bladder injury, especially in cases with previous surgery; followed by exploration, identification, and restoration of normal anatomic relationships. In the Trendelenburg position, the bowel may be packed into the upper abdomen. Both the ureters are traced for pelvic courses till these enter a separate tunnel within the base of the bladder. Dissection of the pararectal space reveals the ureter on its medial margin, as it passes under the uterine artery. Palpation of the ureter between the fingers imparts "clicking" sound. Visible peristalsis is more reliable.

The ureter usually should be dissected away from gynecologic disease process. Placing the tips of a right angle forceps between the adventitial sheath of the ureter and the adjacent tissue to guide the dissection is helpful. If a portion of the ureter is invaded by endometriosis or malignancy, it may have to be resected and ureteroneocystostomy/ureteroureterostomy performed.

The surgeon should always be ureter-conscious to keep it out of harm's way. Care should be taken not only to avoid direct injury and its kinking during obliteration of the cul-de-sac, plication of the uterosacral ligaments, or suspension of the vaginal apex.

Vaginal Approach

In vaginal surgery, we also drain the bladder with a transurethral catheter, and instill undiluted indigo carmine (5 mL)/diluted methylene blue into the bladder. This is done, if the catheter is clamped or removed to keep the dye within the bladder. During surgery, if the bladder is incised, the blue color of the indigo carmine is recognized. The surgeon should avoid a cystotomy by identifying the trigone and base of the bladder. Once the base of the bladder has been dissected free of the lower uterine segment and the vesicoperitoneal fold has been incised, a vaginal retractor should be placed between the bladder and the uterus. This retractor is protective in that it elevates the bladder and lateralizes the ureters. Avoid injury to the bladder with the tip of the refractor.

During vaginal surgery, to palpate the ureters against an appropriately placed vaginal sidewall retractor is very important but difficult in POP. If any doubt about the integrity of the ureters or bladder, cystoscopy should be performed. Dissection of the anterior vaginal wall exposes the urethra and the bladder trigone to injury. Most urethral injuries result from diverticulum repair, anterior colporrhaphy, or instrumentation of the urethra. Some urethral injuries are caused by urethropexy and sling procedures. Urethral injuries, both direct and indirect, may damage the organ's sphincter mechanism and cause SUI.

Laparoscopic Approach

Urinary tract injuries occur in 1–2% of patients who undergo major laparoscopic surgery. Endoscopic adnexectomy poses a higher risk of ureteral injury than does open hysterectomy. Most bladder injuries result from sharp dissection, with or without cautery. During laparoscopy, urinary tract injury may be revealed by direct observation, injection of dye solution, presence of gas in the catheter bag, and detection of bubbles during cystoscopy. If urinary tract injury is suspected, cystoscopy should be performed and sometimes repeated. If ureteral injury is suspected, a ureteral catheter should be inserted.

In summary, the key principles in the repair of acute ureteral injury are as follows:

- Describe questionably viable tissue and stent, if still in doubt
- Strive for a tension-free and watertight anastomosis

- Isolate the repair from infection, retroperitoneal fibrosis, and cancer (use omentum as needed)
- No cancer or radiated tissue should be present at the anastomosis
- Minimize ureteral mobilization
- Ureteral angulations and kinks should be released, if they cause significant obstruction
- Minor ureteral crush injuries may be managed with stenting
- Significant crush injuries require resection of the damaged segment and ureteroneocystostomy or ureteroureterostomy as in cases of complete lacerations of the ureter and loss of a segment
- If there is tension on the anastomosis, it should be relieved by a vesicopsoas hitch procedure or Boari's flap
- If simple repair is not possible and a specialist is not available then divert temporarily

This drain should remain in place until the ureteral catheter has been removed. The ureteral catheter should be left in place for at least 7 days.

Recognition and Management of Bladder Injury

Any injury is recognized by bladder dye instillation, cystoscopy, or cystotomy. The injury site is repaired by 3-0 delayed absorbable sutures in two layers. Postoperative bladder drainage is usually recommended for 10 days in ureter or bladder trauma.

Recognition and Management of Urethral Injury

It is done by catheter insertion or urethroscopy and repaired by 3-0 delayed absorbable sutures or urethroplasty.

Chapter 6

Role of Cystoscopy in Urogynecological Surgery

Suguna Kumar Veera

INTRODUCTION

Due to the anatomic proximity of the urinary and genital tracts, iatrogenic urinary tract injury during pelvic reconstructive surgery and pelvic organ prolapse (POP) repair is a serious complication leading to much morbidity in particular to the formation of genitourinary fistula and the potential loss of renal function, especially if diagnosed postoperatively. The majority of ureteral injuries occur during gynecological operations, and lower urinary tract injury is one of the most common reasons for medical litigation against gynecologists. Incidence of injury to the ureter during gynecologic surgery range from 0.4% to 2.5% and the lower urinary tract injury is higher for some urogynecologic operations.

Intraoperative cystoscopy is safe and allows for immediate recognition and easier repair of injury to lower urinary tract[1] (Fig. 1).

Transurethral cystoscopy is performed using 30 or 70° rigid telescope with 17 French sheaths. A thorough survey of the bladder made with special

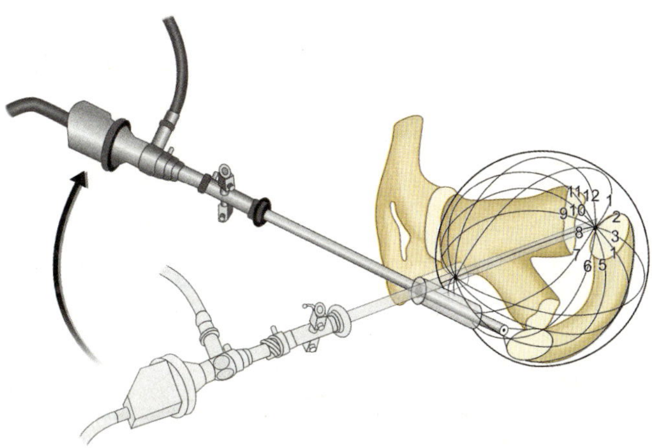

Fig. 1: Cystoscopic sweep.

attention to the portions of the bladder potentially jeopardized by the operative procedure. Inspection of the anterior and the lateral aspects of the mucosa after a midurethral sling or retropubic urethropexy, inspection of the trigone after a difficult vaginal hysterectomy or dissection of a enterocele from the base of the bladder. Assessment of the ureteral integrity after any retropubic dissection, total laparoscopic or robotic hysterectomy, apical support procedures, culdoplasty, colpocleisis, and other complex situations. Whenever there is a suspicion of ureteral injury. Intravenous (IV) administration of indigo carmine 2.5 mL of 0.8% solution approximately 5 minutes before initiating cystoscopy stains the urine blue and facilitates visualization of the ureteral orifices during efflux. Effective alternative to indigo carmine are (a) sodium fluorescein,[2] (b) partial filling the bladder with a solution of either sterile water or 10% dextrose and visualization of the urine stream exiting form the ureteric orifice, (c) administration of IV methylene blue 50 mg over 5 minutes with a small dose of IV furosemide may accelerate the appearance of blue colored urine [methylene blue not to be used in patients on monoamine oxidase (MAO) inhibitors, selective serotonin receptor inhibitors, and selective norepinephrine reuptake inhibitors], and (d) oral phenazopyridine 100–200 mg 30 minutes prior to surgery will color the urine orange.[3]

A 30° *suprapubic cystoscopy* (Fig. 2) with light source and retrograde filling of bladder is an alternative to transurethral cystoscopy for evaluation of lower urinary tract during pelvic surgery with an abdominal approach in supine position. Valuable operative time lost closing the abdominal wound and repositioning to lithotomy position and prepping for transurethral cystoscopy. Also significant cystoscopy finding mandates reopening of the abdomen for surgical correction.

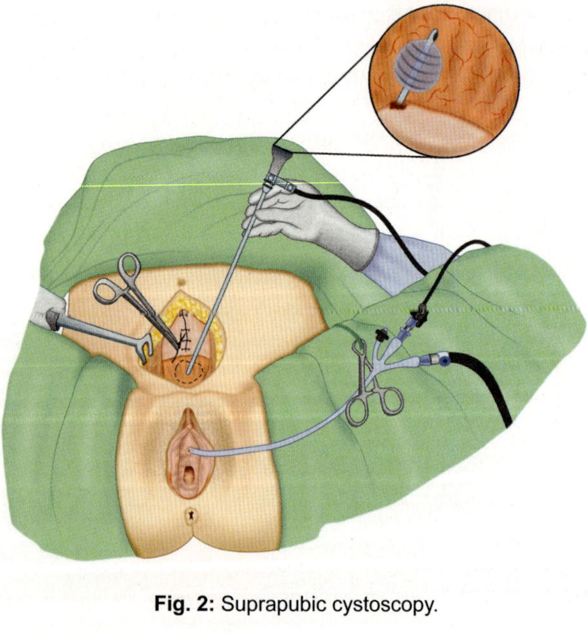

Fig. 2: Suprapubic cystoscopy.

Absence of efflux of urine from ureteral orifices during intraoperative cystoscopy in pelvic surgery is an indication for the passage of ureteral catheter to evaluate for potential obstruction. Vaginal surgery for anterior and or apical POP is associated with intraoperative ureteral obstruction rate of 5.1%. Pre-existing ureteral obstruction requires preoperative assessment of ureters to simplify intraoperative evaluation during complex urogynecological surgery.

URINARY TRACT INJURIES

Iatrogenic injury to bladder occurs from aggressive blunt dissection, sharp dissection, electrocautery, crush injury from retractor, or clamp during pelvic surgery. Bladder injury staged as:[4]

- *Grade 1:* Contusion, intramural hematoma, or partial thickness laceration
- *Grade 2:* Extraperitoneal bladder wall laceration of 2 cm
- *Grade 3:* Extraperitoneal bladder laceration of more than 2 cm or intraperitoneal laceration less than 2 cm
- *Grade 4:* Intraperitoneal laceration of more than 2 cm
- *Grade 5:* Intraperitoneal or extraperitoneal wall laceration involving the trigone or bladder neck.

Ureter injury classified based on the mechanism as laceration, ligation, devascularization, and energy-related. Prompt identification and repair is optimal to avoid postoperative morbidity.[4]

Universal intraoperative cystoscope detected 97.4% of ureteral injuries. It is important to note that a negative cystoscopy result does not guarantee lack of ureteral or bladder injury as there may be partial obstruction or injury with residual patency.[5] Universal intraoperative cystoscopy advised to rule out cystotomy and intravesical suture or mesh placement and to verify bilateral ureteral patency during and after tension-free vaginal tape (TVT) or retropubic mid-urethral sling (MUS), needle urethral suspension, ureter-vaginal fistula repair, and urethral diverticulum. May be indicated in Burch colposuspension, transobturator tape (TOT) or no incision mini sling, pubovaginal slings, POP surgery (anterior and apical). In 70% of the cases the management involves merely removal and replacing the offending suture of closing the cystotomy.

Advantage of intraoperative cystoscopy is early diagnosis of bladder and ureter injury to avoid additional surgery and the development of urinary fistula and possible loss of renal function. Diagnosis of other pathology cancer, fetal blood (FB), and congenital anomaly.

Disadvantage is the time, cost, and urinary tract infection (UTI), prophylactic antibiotic for the surgery will probably cover.

Although routine cystoscopy clearly increases the intraoperative detection rate of urinary tract injuries. The systemic review of 79 mostly retrospective studies shows that it does not appear to have much effect on the part of injury detection rate. The estimated postoperative ureteric injury detection rate per 1,000 surgeries were 1.6 without routine cystoscopy and 0.7 with routine cystoscopy and postoperative bladder injury detection rate of 0.8 without routine cystoscopy and 1.0 with routine cystoscopy.[6]

Most but not all lower urinary tract injuries can be detected by intraoperative cystoscopy. Published data suggest a sensitivity of 80–90% (Level A). Intraoperative cystoscopy detects most unsuspected injury (Level B), thus routine cystoscopy recommended at the time of laparoscopic hysterectomy and urogynecological surgery (Level B).

REFERENCES

1. Kwon CH, Goldberg RP, Koduri S, et al. The use of intraoperative cystoscopy in major vaginal and urogynecologic surgeries. . Am J Obst Gynecol. 2002;187(6):1466-71.
2. Doyle P J, Lipetskaia L, Duocy E, et al. Sodium fluorescein use during intraoperative cystoscopy. Obst Gynecol. 2015;125(3):548-50.
3. Barbieri RL. Farewell to indigo carmine. OBG Manag. 2014; 26(9):8-9.
4. Delacroix SE Jr, Winters JC. Urinary tract injuries: recognition and management. Clin Colon Rectal Surg. 2010;23(2):104-12.
5. Donald V Maathai. E, Chatwani A, et al. Accuracy of cystoscope in the diagnosis of ureteral injury in the benign gynecological surgery. Int Urogynecol J Pelvic Floor Dysfunct. 2003;14:427-31.
6. Teeluckdharry B, Glimour D, Flowerdew G. Urinary tract injury at benign gynecological surgery and the role of cystoscopy: a systematic review and meta-analysis. Obstet Gynecol. 2015;126(6):1161-9.

Chapter 7

Update in Pharmacotherapy for Female Urinary Incontinence

Harsha Ananthram, Jay Iyer, Ajay Rane

INTRODUCTION

Urinary incontinence (UI) is defined by the International Continence Society as "the complaint of any involuntary leakage of urine". UI may occur as a result of a number of abnormalities of function of the lower urinary tract or as a result of other illnesses, which tend to cause leakage in different situations.

Urinary incontinence affects the physical, psychological and social well-being of older people, and is a major cause of admission to residential aged care. The incidence increases with age. UI is not a normal part of aging. It is the loss of urine control due to a combination of genitourinary pathology, age-related changes, comorbid conditions and environmental obstacles[1] (Table 1).

Table 1: Classification of urinary incontinence in women.[2]

Type	*Pathophysiology*	*Symptoms*	*Patient profile*
Most common			
Urge (UUI)	❑ Detrusor overactivity ❑ Neurologic disorders ❑ Spinal cord injury	Loss of urine accompanied or preceded by strong desire to void; may be accompanied by frequency and nocturia	❑ Most common in older adults ❑ Strong association with stroke
Stress (SUI)	❑ Increased urethral mobility ❑ Intrinsic sphincter dysfunction	Loss of urine with physical exertion or increases in intra-abdominal pressure (e.g. sneezing, coughing, laughing)	❑ Most common in younger women ❑ Second most common type in older women
Mixed (MUI)	Mixed etiology	Combination of urge and stress symptoms	Overall most common type

Contd...

Contd...

Type	*Pathophysiology*	*Symptoms*	*Patient profile*
Less common			
Overflow	Anatomic obstruction Impaired detrusor contractility from neurologic disorders, including diabetic neuropathy	Dribbling and/or continuous leakage associated with incomplete bladder emptying	Bladder outlet obstruction is uncommon in women More often occurs because of neurologic disorders

(UUI: Urge urinary incontinence; SUI: Stress urinary incontinence; MUI: Mixed urinary incontinence).

ASSESSMENT AND TRIAGE

Assessment of women prior to initiating treatment involves determination of the type of UI and its severity. While most women with incontinence will have improved symptoms with therapy, some do not achieve full continence. Thus, treatment should proceed in a stepwise fashion with a patient-centered emphasis on improving quality of life. Chronic exposure to urine can result in contact dermatitis and skin breakdown resulting from chronic irritation—it needs to be addressed by frequent pad changes and topical creams and ointments. The focus needs to be not just on the symptom being considered but on the patient.

An initial assessment of symptom severity includes urine dipstick and microscopy or sensitivity testing and bladder diary recordings (for a minimum of 3 days) that cover variations in usual activities, voiding frequency patterns, fluid input/output and bladder volumes. A voiding diary can also give an objective assessment of severity and may be helpful in assessing impact of treatment.

Tools that patients complete such as the pelvic floor distress inventory, Pelvic Floor impact questionnaire, and Overactive Bladder Questionnaire help focus treatment goals and evaluate treatment efficacy; these should be considered part of the baseline assessment.

A good history that is elicited along with information from patient questionnaires will help optimize medical conditions and medications that could act as contributory factors to the symptoms of UI.

STEPWISE APPROACH

The initial treatment of UI includes lifestyle modifications and pelvic floor muscle exercise for all patients with UI along with bladder training in women with urgency incontinence.

Lifestyle interventions include changing the amount of fluid ingested, smoking cessation, reduction in caffeine consumption and the avoidance of over-restricting fluid intake that could lead to worsening urgency and constipation. Eating foods with dietary fiber that help to regulate the bowels and to avoid constipation is also recommended for bladder health.[3]

Dietary advice and physical activity must be recommended as part of a weight loss regimen for women with a body mass index (BMI) equal to and greater than 30, to help reduce the number of incontinence episodes[4] with a greater benefit seen for stress than urge UI.

Pelvic floor exercises (PFE), as taught by physiotherapists, strengthen the pelvic floor musculature to provide a backboard for the urethra to compress on and to reflexively inhibit detrusor contractions.

Biofeedback as a supplement to pelvic muscle exercises is particularly useful in women who are unable to properly isolate the pelvic floor or use accessory muscles during pelvic floor contractions. This modality involves placement of a vaginal pressure sensor within the vagina that measures pressure and provides an audible or visual feedback of strength of pelvic floor contraction.

Behavioral therapy options including timed voiding, habit retraining, prompted voiding and bladder retraining have different methods and outcomes. Timed voiding includes using a fixed toileting schedule. Habit retraining uses information from the bladder diary to design a toileting schedule around pre-empting UI episodes. Prompted voiding involves monitoring the older adult's voiding pattern to prompt them to use the toilet and giving social reinforcement. Bladder retraining with urgency suppression involves lengthening the interval between voiding.

PHARMACOLOGIC THERAPY

Stress urinary incontinence (SUI): Medications are used selectively in the treatment of SUI and not as first-line treatment.

Vaginal estrogen preparations should be considered as adjuncts to first-line management with PFE. Improved continence has been noted[5] in women as atrophic symptoms such as dysuria, frequency and SUI are ameliorated by its use.

Midodrine is an alpha-adrenergic receptor agonist that has been used in mild-to-moderate SUI. Potential adverse effects of this class include hypertension, dry mouth, nausea, and insomnia. In combination with estrogen, it shows an increased efficacy compared with monotherapy with regard to symptom relief.[6]

Duloxetine is a serotonin–norepinephrine reuptake inhibitor (SNRI) that has, for SUI, shown a reduction in incontinence episodes and an improved quality of life. Common side effects include nausea, headache, constipation, dry mouth, and insomnia. Duloxetine is effective in patients who may suffer from associated depression but are otherwise more sparingly used as the preferred treatment option for SUI after PFE and surgery.

Urge urinary incontinence (UUI): The main pharmacological treatment options for UUI are antimuscarinic agents such as oxybutynin, tolterodine, trospium, solifenacin, darifenacin, and fesoterodine. In a recent meta-analysis compiling data regarding "trade-offs" between efficacy and side-effect profiles, authors concluded that 40 mg/day trospium, 100 mg/g per day oxybutynin gel, and 4 mg/day fesoterodine were the most favorable formulations.[7] However, acceptance of clear superiority of one antimuscarinic over another is lacking.

Improvement in symptoms may take up to 4 weeks, and it may take up to 12 weeks for medications to have full efficacy.

Adverse effects of these agents include dry mouth, constipation, headache, dry eyes, blurred vision, tachycardia, sedation and cognitive impairment in elderly patients. They are contraindicated in patients with narrow-angle glaucoma, impaired gastric emptying or urinary retention.

It is good practice to commence at the lowest dose and titrate up as needed after 2 weeks if the patient has insufficient response and thus minimize the side effects.

The first new class of medications for the treatment of UUI in over 30 years, mirabegron, a beta-3 agonist, was Food and Drug Administration approved for overactive bladder in June 2012. In contrast to antimuscarinics, this class of drugs target the beta-3 receptors in the bladder dome that promote detrusor relaxation. Adverse effects of mirabegron include hypertension, urinary tract infections, headaches, and nasopharyngitis. The medication is contraindicated in patients with urinary retention or uncontrolled hypertension.

In patients who are taking mirabegron with an antimuscarinic, it would be advisable to monitor for urinary retention by measuring postvoid residual volumes by a follow-up visit in 4 weeks or if new voiding dysfunction symptoms arise.

THIRD-LINE THERAPY

Botulinum toxin A (BTX-A), a serotype of the neurotoxin produced by *Clostridium botulinum*, is increasingly utilized as a safe and effective treatment option for refractory overactive bladder, blocks acetylcholine release at presynaptic neuromuscular junctions, thereby decreasing detrusor overactivity and incontinence. It is additionally believed to alter urothelial sensory afferent pathways and help alleviate hypersensitivity responses, an explanation as why BTX-A is also effective in decreasing urinary urgency and frequency, and increasing bladder capacity.[8]

With BTX-A use, important contraindications or considerations remain—current urinary tract infection, malignancy, obstruction, pregnancy and neuromuscular junction disorders such as myasthenia gravis (autoantibodies to acetylcholine receptors) and Lambert-Eaton syndrome (failure of nerves to release acetylcholine).

Sacral nerve stimulation consists of a lead wire with four electrodes that are positioned along the sacral nerve roots—most commonly S3. This is then attached to an implantable pulse generator (IPG) that is surgically placed in the upper buttocks and provides non-painful electrical stimulation. Procedurally, this involves a two-step process [either in office percutaneous nerve evaluation (PNE) or stage I in the operating room] where the patient can test the efficacy (reduction in symptoms >50%) prior to final IPG placement.[9]

CONCLUSION

Management of UI should commence only after a comprehensive assessment and exploration of the preferences for treatment have been completed.

The principles involved in management of patients with UI, to achieve optimal results, include a broad understanding of the pathophysiology involved, a stepwise approach from conservative options to more invasive therapies, setting realistic patient expectations by emphasizing symptom reduction over cure and a focus follow-up visits to assess progress and satisfaction level.

REFERENCES

1. Royal Australian College of General Practitioners. Medical care of older persons in residential aged care facilities, 4th edition. South Melbourne: Royal Australian College of General Practitioners; 2006.
2. Hersh L, Salzman B. Clinical management of urinary incontinence in women. Am Fam Physician. 2013;87(9):634-40.
3. Kaplan SA, Dmochowski R, Cash BD, et al. Systematic review of the relationship between bladder and bowel function: implications for patient management. Int J Clin Pract. 2013;67(3):205-16.
4. Moore K, Dumoulin C, Bradley C, et al. Adult conservative management. In: Abrams P, Cardozo L, Khoury S, Wein A (Eds). Incontinence: Proceedings from the 5th International Consultation on Incontinence. Plymouth, UK: Health Publications; 2013. pp. 1103-1228.
5. Cody JD, Jacobs ML, Richardson K, et al. Oestrogen therapy for urinary incontinence in post-menopausal women. Cochrane Database Syst Rev. 2012;10:CD001405.
6. Rovner ES, Wyman J, Lam S. Urinary incontinence. In: DiPiro JT, Talbert RL, Yee GC, Matzke GR, Wells BG, Posey LM. (Eds). Pharmacotherapy: A Pathophysiologic Approach, 9th edition. New York, NY: McGraw-Hill; 2014.
7. Buser N, Ivic S, Kessler TM, et al. Efficacy and adverse events of antimuscarinics for treating overactive bladder: network meta-analyses. Eur Urol. 2012;62:1040-60.
8. Schmid DM, Sauermann P, Werner M, et al. Experience with 100 cases treated with botulinum-A toxin injections in the detrusor muscle for idiopathic overactive bladder syndrome refractory to anticholinergics. J Urol. 2006;176:177-85.
9. Gormley EA, Lightner DJ, Faraday M, et al. American Urological Association, Society of Urodynamics, Female Pelvic Medicine Diagnosis and treatment of overactive bladder (non-neurogenic) in adults: AUA/SUFU guideline amendment. J Urol. 2015;193(5):1572.

Chapter 8

The use of Botox in the Management of Overactive Bladder

Jagdish Gandhi

INTRODUCTION

Botulinum toxin (BOTOX) is a potent neurotoxin derived from Gram-positive anaerobic spore-forming organism, *Clostridium Botulinum*. Type A (BOTOX) is currently used for the management of overactive bladder symptoms caused by detrusor overactivity and for the patients who have not responded to the conservative management. Now there are several evidences to support its use for patient with overactive bladder (OAB) symptoms. Adverse events are only few and serious events are rare. The operative procedure is simple using a cystoscope. The beneficial effect of BOTOX would last up to 6–9 months and a repeat injection may be necessary.

INDICATIONS

Botox was initially used in the spinal cord injury patients with detrusor sphincter dyssynergia. More recently it is used in the management of:

- Neurogenic detrusor over-activity
- Idiopathic detrusor over-activity
- Dysfunctional voiding
- Pelvic pain.

The aim of this article is to:

- Overview the current management of overactive bladder
- Describe mechanism of action of BOTOX
- Describe preoperative actions and operative technique
- Discuss efficacy and potential risks of use of intravesical BOTOX
- Review current recommendations and guidelines.

MANAGEMENT

Management of OAB in Women (Specialized Management)

The ICI guidelines.[1] Management of OAB in women has been described in the Flowchart 1.

Flowchart 1: Management of OAB in women.

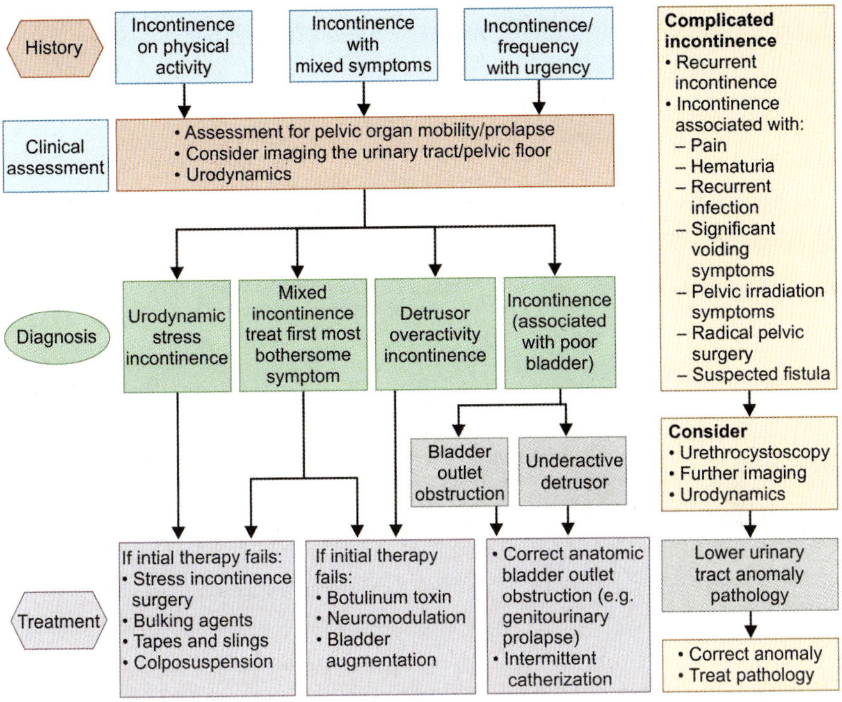

MECHANISM OF ACTION OF BOTOX

Seven serotypes A to G have been identified. However, two types, A and B are available for clinical use. Currently in UK, 2 preparations of Botulinum toxin A are available - BOTOX (Allergan Ltd) and Dysport (Ipsen Ltd).[2] Most studies and meta-analysis are from the use of BOTOX.

The physiological action of botulinum toxin A is probably only effective in women where detrusor overactivity is the cause of their OAB. It is believed that when it is injected into the walls of the bladder, it paralyses the detrusor muscle so that it is no longer contracts involuntarily.[2] (Flowchart 2) The clinical effect begins within 1-3 weeks and the benefit lasts for 6–9 months. BOTOX thus provides durable yet reversible treatment option for detrusor overactivity. Repeat injection may be required.

Preoperative Management

- Patients require accurate, relevant and digestible information to make informed decisions about their treatment
- Explain possible voiding disorder and need for self-catheterization and the process involved. Patient should be willing and able to perform self-catheterization
- Rule out urinary infections

Flowchart 2: Mechanism of action of BOTOX.[3,4]

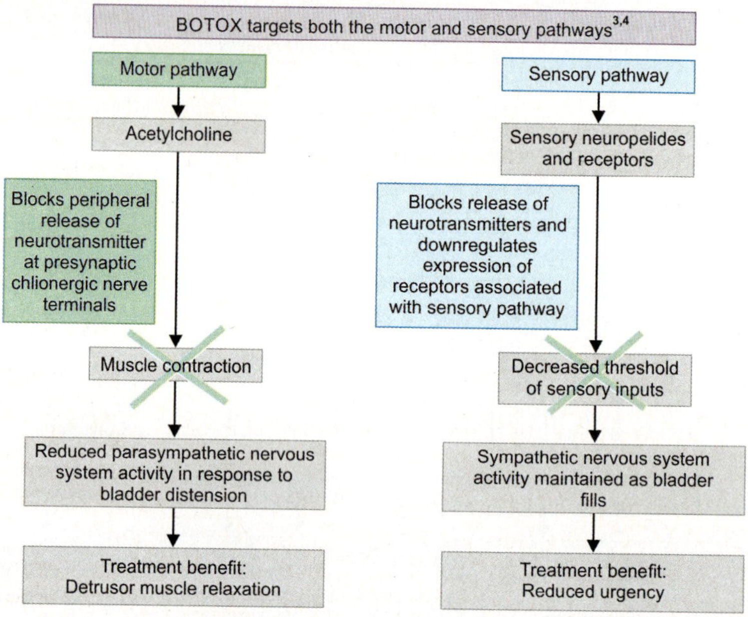

- Contraindications include pregnancy, myasthenia gravis, bladder malignancy, and bleeding disorders
- Patients on anticoagulant therapy need to be managed appropriately to decrease the risk of bleeding
- Appropriate prophylactic antibiotics should be administered.

BOTOX Injection Technique

The intravesical BOTOX can be administered under general anesthesia or local anesthesia using either rigid or flexible cystoscope. 100–200 units of BOTOX are mixed in 20 mL of normal saline without shaking the vial. It is then injected into the detrusor muscles at 20 separate sites, sparing the trigone and ureteric ostia so as to avoid vesicoureteric reflux (Fig. 1). Patients should be observed for at least 30 minutes post-injection. Patients must have a spontaneous void before leaving.

Postoperative review at four weeks is recommended to ensure complete emptying of the bladder. Signs of UTI, hematuria and voiding difficulties need to be monitored.

Efficacy and Tolerability of Intravesical BOTOX

In recent years there have been a number of publications to support efficacy and safety of BOTOX. Three systemic reviews with the data from 1320 patients, including some placebo-controlled trials, have been published. These show a significant decrease in mean number of urinary incontinence episodes per day

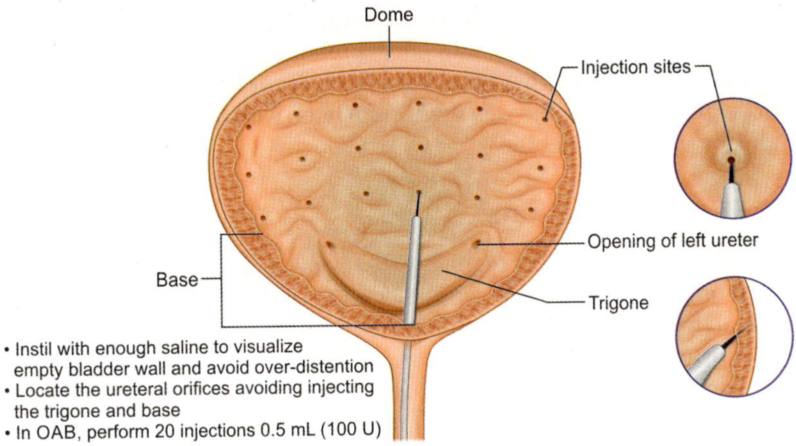

Fig. 1: Intravesical BOTOX® injection technique.[5,6]

by 2.77 compared with 1 after placebo. Similarly mean numbers of micturitions per day also reduced by 1.61 as compared to 0.87 after placebo.[7-10]

BOTOX significantly improved all OAB symptoms in patients who had an inadequate response to anticholinergic therapy. BOTOX significantly improved QoL vs placebo. Most patients (93%) did not require CIC.[5]

The most recent trials have shown that 100 units may be as effective as 200 units but with a lower rate of adverse events and a lower rate of urinary retention.[5,6,11]

There are several evidences that repeated injections are equally effective in terms of urinary frequency, urgency and incontinence, and quality of life assessments.[12]

Adverse Effects of BOTOX

- Most common adverse events are urinary tract infection and dysuria (Table 1)
- Flu-like syndrome has been reported

Table 1: Adverse effects of BOTOX.

Adverse event ≥3%, N (%)	*First 12 weeks*		*Any time in treatment cycle 1*	
	BOTOX® 100 U (N = 552)	*Placebo (N = 542)*	*BOTOX® 100 U (N = 552)*	*Placebo (N = 542)*
Urinary tract infection	99 (17.9)	30 (5.5)	141 (25.5)	52 (9.6)
Dysuria	50 (9.1)	36 (6.6)	60 (10.9)	38 (7.0)
Urinary retention	31 (5.6)	2 (0.4)	32 (5.8)	2 (0.4)
Bacteriuria	24 (4.3)	11 (2.0)	44 (8.0)	19 (3.5)
Pollakiuria (Frequency)	9 (1.6)	4 (0.7)	11 (2.0)	5 (0.9)
Residual urine volume	17 (3.1)	1 (0.2)	19 (3.4)	2 (0.4)

- Transient muscular weakness in the extremities has been reported
- Systemic effects are rare. Side effects related to spread of toxin distant from the site of administration have been reported, sometimes resulting in death, which in some cases was associated with dysphagia, pneumonia and/or significant debility.

NICE Recommendations[2]

- After a multidisciplinary team (MDT) review, offer bladder wall injection with botulinum toxin A to women with OAB caused by proven detrusor overactivity that has not responded to conservative management (including OAB drug therapy).
- Discuss the risks and benefits of treatment with botulinum toxin A with women before seeking informed consent, covering:
  - The likelihood of being symptom free or having a large reduction in symptoms
  - The risk of clean intermittent catheterization and the potential for it to be needed for variable lengths of time after the effect of the injections has worn off
  - The absence of evidence on duration of effect between treatments and the long-term efficacy and risks
  - The risk of adverse effects, including an increased risk of urinary tract infection.
- Start treatment with botulinum toxin A only if women:
  - Have been trained in clean intermittent catheterization and have performed the technique successfully, and
  - Are able and willing to perform clean intermittent catheterization on a regular basis for as long as needed.
- Use 200 units when offering botulinum toxin A.
- Consider 100 units of botulinum toxin A for women who would prefer a dose with a lower chance of catheterization and accept a reduced chance of success.
- If the first botulinum toxin A treatment has no effect discuss with the MDT.
- If botulinum toxin A treatment is effective, offer follow-up at 6 months or sooner if symptoms return for repeat treatment without an MDT referral.

CONCLUSION

Botulinum toxin A (BOTOX) is a potent neurotoxin used for the management of idiopathic detrusor overactivity. It is believed that when it is injected into the walls of the bladder, it paralyses the detrusor muscle so that it is no longer contracts involuntarily.

NICE, UK recommends full counseling of the patients prior to BOTOX administration. BOTOX 100–200 units is injected into the detrusor muscles at 20 separate sites using a cystoscope under local or general anesthesia.

BOTOX significantly improves all OAB symptoms, reduces urinary incontinence episodes and frequency of micturition. Most common adverse events are urinary tract infection and dysuria. The clinical effect begins within 1–3 weeks and the benefit lasts for 6–9 months. Repeat injection may be required.

REFERENCES

1. Abrams P, Cardozo L, S Khoury et al. (Eds). Incontinence: 5th Edition, 2013;ISBN:978-9953-493-21-3.
2. National Institute for Health and Care Excellence. Urinary incontinence in women: the management of urinary incontinence in women. (Clinical guideline 171.) 2013. http://guidance.nice.org.uk/CG171.
3. Purves D, Augustine GJ, Fitzpatrick D, et al. Autonomic regulation of the bladder. neuroscience, 2nd edition, 2001.
4. Apostolidis A, Dasgupta P, Fowler CJ. Proposed mechanism for the efficacy of injected botulinum toxin in the treatment of human detrusor overactivity. Eur Urol. 2006;49:644-50.
5. Chapple C, Sievert KD, MacDiarmid S, et al. Onabotulinumtoxin A 100 U significantly improves all idiopathic overactive bladder symptoms and quality of life in patients with overactive bladder and urinary incontinence: a randomised, double-blind, placebo-controlled trial. Eur Urol. 2013;64:249-56.
6. Nitti VW, Dmochowski R, Herschorn S, et al. Onabotulinumtoxin A for the treatment of patients with overactive bladder and urinary incontinence: results of a phase 3, randomized, placebo controlled trial. J Urol. 2013;189:2186-93.
7. Mangera A, Andersson KE, Apostolidis A, et al. Contemporary management of lower urinary tract disease with botulinum toxin A: a systematic review of Botox (onabotulinumtoxin A) and Dysport (abobotulinumtoxin A). Eur Urol. 2011;60:784-95.
8. Mangera A, Apostolidis A, Andersson KE, et al. An updated systematic review and statistical comparison of standardised mean outcomes for the use of botulinum toxin in the management of lower urinary tract disorders. Eur Urol. 2014;65:981-90.
9. Anger JT, Weinberg A, Suttorp MJ, et al. Outcomes of intravesical botulinum toxin for idiopathic overactive bladder symptoms: a systematic review of the literature. J Urol. 2010;183:2258-64.
10. Cui Y, Wang L, Liu L, et al. Botulinum toxin-A injections for idiopathic overactive bladder: a systematic review and meta-analysis. Urol Int. 2013;91:429-38.
11. Denys P, Le NL, Ghout I, et al. Efficacy and safety of low doses of onabotulinumtoxin A for the treatment of refractory idiopathic overactive bladder: a multicentre, double-blind, randomised, placebo-controlled dose-ranging study. Eur Urol. 2012;61:520-9.
12. Sahai A, Dowson C, Khan MS, Dasgupta P. Repeated injections of botulinum toxin-a for idiopathic detrusor overactivity. Urology. 2010;75:552-8.

Chapter 9

Pelvic Organ Prolapse

A Tamilselvi

INTRODUCTION

Pelvic organ prolapse (POP) can affect women of all age-groups and is a common problem. The lifetime risk of undergoing an operation for POP is estimated to be around 11%. With increase in life expectancy the number of women presenting with POP is likely to increase in future. POP is not a life-threatening condition but can significantly impair the quality of life of the individual.

Many risk factors can lead to POP such as prolonged labor, instrumental delivery, multiparity, obesity, physical labor over many years and genetic and familial predisposition. However, usually there is very little women can do to reduce the impact of these risk factors.

Assessment of POP includes identification of defect in all the three vaginal compartments—apical, anterior, and posterior. The three levels of endopelvic fascia support described by DeLancey, explains failure of specific aspects of the fascia in each of these compartments. Apical compartment prolapse results from failure of the uterosacral and cardinal ligament complex. The anterior compartment prolapse (cystocele) and posterior compartment prolapse (rectocele) result from defects in the pubocervical and rectovaginal endopelvic fascia respectively.

Prolapse symptoms can include dragging sensation or heaviness in the vagina, backache, a sensation of lump in the vagina, which may be associated with bladder, bowel or sexual dysfunction. Objective assessment of POP includes staging using either the Baden-Walker or POP quantification system. No specific investigation is needed in the diagnosis of POP. Examination helps in identifying the compartments of prolapse, associated pelvic mass, atrophic changes or other pelvic pathology.

Management of POP is two-fold: either conservative or surgical. Conservative measures play a significant role in the management of POP. This includes lifestyle interventions, pelvic floor exercises and pessaries. Surgical option is the presumed definitive management in prolapse.

The choice of type of surgery depends on several factors such as the age of the patient, pre-existing comorbid problems, site of prolapse, route of repair and the surgeon preference for a particular technique. Depending on the compartment of prolapse, the surgical techniques can be discussed.

APICAL PROLAPSE (UTEROVAGINAL AND VAULT)

Apical prolapse (uterovaginal prolapse) in an unmarried young girl, commonly results from congenital weakness of the pelvic supports. The various sling surgeries, Purandrare's, Khanna's and Virkud's composite slings are some of the procedures which are helpful in managing this condition.

In a reproductive aged woman, whether the uterus is to be retained needs to be decided. The age of the patient, desire for preservation of fertility and future pregnancies, presence of precancerous lesions or other pelvic pathology can influence the decision regarding uterine conservation. In general, removal of uterus appears to improve access for a complete pelvic floor reconstruction.

In most parts of the world, surgical treatment of uterovaginal prolapse is the traditional vaginal hysterectomy (VH) with or without anterior and posterior repair. Combining this with plication of the uterosacral ligaments (McCall culdoplasty) or high uterosacral ligament suspension (HULS) recreates vaginal apex support.

Culdoplasty technique usually involves placement of internal and external sutures on the uterosacral ligament after hysterectomy and plicating them in the midline and incorporating the peritoneum in between. This obliterates the cul-de-sac and reduces the risk of postoperative enterocele.

High uterosacral ligament suspension procedure can be employed for vault support either at the end of the hysterectomy or for vaginal vault prolapse. In HULS, the uterosacral ligament portion, proximal to the ischial spine is used to suspend the vaginal apex along with incorporation of the anterior and posterior vaginal walls to create a pericervical ring.

In the management of vault prolapse, one of the most common vaginal procedures employed is sacrospinous ligament suspension (SSLS). The procedure aims to suspend the vault to the sacrospinous ligament. Sutures are placed on the sacrospinous ligament and are secured to the vaginal vault, either at the end of the vaginal hysterectomy to suspend the vault or in the management of vault prolapse.

Using the abdominal approach, the apical prolapse can be addressed using abdominal sacrocolpopexy (ASCP). In ASCP the vault is secured to the anterior surface of sacrum at the level of S1-S2 by a graft material. Usually, it is done as an open technique, but recently is also being performed using laparoscopic and robotic approaches. Several studies have confirmed a good long-term success rate with ASCP ranging from 77%–100% for the apical compartment. It is considered a durable technique for apical prolapse repair. In ASCP there is better anatomical restoration of the vaginal axis and the vaginal configuration is maintained.

UTERUS PRESERVING SURGERIES

Hysterectomy as a component of prolapse repair may not be preferred by some women with prolapse. The fact that the uterus is not the cause but rather the effect in uterine prolapse has been clearly defined with anatomical studies. Abdominal sacrohysteropexy, abdominal uterosacral suspension, sacrospinous hysteropexy, and Manchester procedure are some of the commonly employed procedures in uterine preservation.

ANTERIOR AND POSTERIOR WALL POP (CYSTOCELE AND RECTOCELE) REPAIR

Both anterior and posterior vaginal wall defects very rarely occur in isolation. Thorough pelvic floor examination is essential, to determine whether there is coexistent prolapse of other sites. When prolapse is present at more than one anatomic site, a coordinated approach to the repair may be required. The repair outcomes have been shown to be significantly improved when performed concurrently with an apical support repair. In cystocele repair (anterior wall), anterior colporrhaphy and vaginal or abdominal paravaginal repair, addresses the native tissue defects to provide support. In rectocele (posterior compartment) repair traditional posterior colporrhaphy and site-specific repair are the two main methods of transvaginal rectocele repair, both with comparative outcomes. With the Food and Drug Administration (FDA) regulation on use of mesh and mesh kite, augmenting the anterior and posterior vaginal wall with these techniques are not in common use.

CONCLUSION

In any patient presenting with POP there are varied surgical options available. There are patient factors which can determine the route and technique such as age, associated comorbid factors or other pelvic pathology. In addition, the surgeon's training and experience can also influence this decision making process. It is therefore essential for the pelvic surgeon to be skillful in the different surgical techniques.

Chapter 10

Role of Urodynamic Study in Stress Urinary Incontinence

Anju Soni

INTRODUCTION

Stress urinary incontinence (SUI) is a condition of involuntary loss of urine on effort, physical exertion, sneezing or coughing that is often, bothersome to the patient and frequently affects the quality of life. The evaluation in women with symptoms of SUI includes the following steps:

The purpose of history taking is to determine the type of urinary incontinence (UI) that is bothersome to the patients. UI is commonly classified as stress, urge, postural continuous (or total), insensible (spontaneous), coital, or incontinence associated with chronic urinary retention (previously referred to as overflow incontinence), nocturnal enuresis or some combination thereof. The history should include questions about the type of incontinence (e.g. stress, urge, mixed), precipitating events, frequency of occurrence, severity, pad use, and effect of symptoms on activities of daily living.

Questions should be asked to assess symptoms related to bladder storage and emptying functions. Storage symptoms include frequency, nocturia, urgency and incontinence. Emptying or voiding symptoms include hesitancy, slow stream, intermittency, straining to void, spraying of urinary stream, feeling of incomplete emptying, need to immediately revoid, postmicturition leakage, position-dependent micturition and dysuria. Health care providers can use validated questionnaires to evaluate bother, severity and the relative contribution of urge UI and SUI symptoms. Patients with uncomplicated SUI will have classic symptoms of leakage on effort or physical exertion. In contrast, inability to reach the toilet which is associated with urgency indicates the presence of urge UI.

Urodynamic investigations are an essential component in the management of women who present with lower urinary tract symptoms. The understanding helps to equip individuals with the knowledge and skills required to use urodynamic investigations within the clinical context. Once trained, a clinician should be able to:

- Undertake an appropriate urogynecological clinical evaluation
- Select the optimum urodynamic investigations for individual patients

- Perform all relevant urodynamic investigations
- Establish a diagnosis and formulate a treatment plan
- Effectively communicate the above information to the patient and colleagues.

URODYNAMIC STUDIES

Surgical correction of incontinence is invasive and not without risk. However, the "bladder is an unreliable witness," and historical information may not always accurately indicate the true underlying type of incontinence. Thus, if initial conservative management is unsuccessful or surgical treatment is anticipated then, objective assessment is pursued. In addition, if symptoms and physical findings are incongruous then, objective urodynamic studies (UDS) using simple or multichannel cystometrics may also be indicated. For example, in a woman with mixed urinary incontinence who has symptoms of both stress and urge urinary incontinence, UDS may reveal that only the urgency component is responsible for her incontinence. These cases are treated with behavioral, physical and/or pharmacologic therapy initially. Thus, if identified by UDS, these individuals can avoid unnecessary surgery. Additionally, surgical therapy may be modified if UDS reveals parameters consistent with intrinsic sphincter deficiency (ISD).

Despite these indications, UDS remains controversial. Leakage noted during testing is not always clinically relevant. In addition, testing may be uninformative if the original of ending maneuver or situation that led to incontinence cannot be reproduced during testing. Moreover, objective confirmation of the diagnosis is not always necessary since, empiric nonsurgical therapy in women with urgency predominant UI undergoing surgical treatment, the outcomes were no different 1 year later as in those screened by urodynamic studies, compared with those evaluated by a simple office evaluation. The office testing included demonstrable leakage during examination, urine analysis without infection and postvoid residual (PVR) urine volume less than150 mL.

The urodynamic investigation was developed as an aid to diagnosis in patients with the history of lower urinary tract symptoms. The urodynamic team encompasses a number of varied physiological tests of bladder and urethral function, which aim to demonstrate an underlying abnormality of storage or voiding.

The battery of tests includes simple cystometry, multichannel cystometry, ambulatory urodynamics, uroflowmetry as well as various other tests for urethral function. Filling and voiding cystometry is the most commonly performed test. This involves placement of fluid- filled or solid-state pressure transducers into the bladder and rectum and together with a fine catheter to fill the bladder artificially. During the filling phase, observations are made of any detrusor contractions, bladder sensation and compliance and any fluid leakage, either spontaneous or on provocation. During the voiding phase, the maximum urinary flow as well as voided volume and timing are measured.

Much progress has been made in recent years with clear definitions and standardization from International Continence Society. Currently therefore, it is possible to differentiate between SUI and overactive bladder (OAB) by urodynamics. Urodynamic findings do correlate with patient symptoms and thus, with a reasonable accuracy. Overall, the sensitivity is 0.82, 0.69 and 0.51 for stress urgency and mixed urinary incontinence, respectively. However, there is no reliable evidence that shows that urodynamics influences operative outcome. The validity and clinical usefulness of ureteral pressure assessment remains controversial. Similarly, urodynamics to reveal occult SUI in patients with pelvic organ prolapse needs standardization of the reducing maneuvers.

Recent recommendations from NICE1, UK includes not to perform multichannel cystometry before starting conservative management. It is though indicated before the surgery, if patient has symptoms of OAB voiding dysfunction, anterior compartment prolapse or had a previous surgery for stress incontinence. NICE recommends not performing cystometry in a small group of women with clear diagnosis of SUI on history and clinical examination.

Preoperative multichannel urodynamic testing is not necessary before planning primary anti-incontinence surgery in women, with uncomplicated SUI. As indicated by observed urinary leakage from the urethra by provocative stress, measured a normal urinalysis result (without urinary tract infection), no POP beyond the hymen and a normal postvoid residual urine volume. Randomized controlled trial results have demonstrated that in women with uncomplicated SUI, the outcome 1 year after midurethral sling surgery were the same for those who had a basic office assessment performance by trained pelvic floor health care providers compared with those, who had a preoperative evaluation that included urodynamic testing. However, women who have complicated SUI may benefit from multichannel urodynamic testing and other diagnostic tests before initiation of treatment, especially surgery. Determination of the need for additional diagnostic tests, surgery should be based on clinical judgment after completion of the basic UI evolution, outlined in this document. Clinical judgment should guide the health care provider's decision to preoperative multichannel urodynamic testing or to refer the patient to a specialist with appropriate training and experience in female pelvic medical and reconstructive surgery.

However, diagnosis were changed in some patients who underwent UDS as the surgeons were more likely, to diagnose ISD and less likely to diagnose OAB, suggesting that UDS did change the clinician's diagnosis before surgery.

Chapter 11

Urinary Tract Injury During Urogynecological Surgery: Prevention and Management

Vineet Mishra

INTRODUCTION

Urogynecology, the evolving sub branch of gynaecology has revolutionized the management of various urogynecological conditions over the past few decades. Since, the urinary tract (UT) is closely related to the genital tract, it becomes indispensable for a gynecologist to have a thorough knowledge of the anatomy of the urinary tract and the possible urinary tract injury that could be encountered during gynecological surgery. It is estimated that 52%–82% of iatrogenic urinary tract injuries occur during gynecologic surgery.[1] Let us have an overview of the possible urinary tract injuries during the urogynecological surgeries and their prevention and management.

SURGERY FOR PROLAPSE

Vaginal Hysterectomy

Injury to the urinary tract (UT) during vaginal hysterectomy (VH) most often involves the urinary bladder rather than the ureter. However, ureteric injury do can happen. The rate of ureteral injury for vaginal hysterectomy is 0.2 injuries per 1,000 cases.[1]

Ureteric Injury

Patients with grade IV cystocele and procidentia can have extremely thin and dilated ureters that can be enclosed in the prolapse and thus predisposed to ureteral injury. Majority of the ureteral injury are during vaginal vault closure where the ureter can get ligated or get kinked by displacement.[2]

In case of VH, the primary risk point is the clamping and ligation of the cardinal ligament. As the cervix is pulled down through the vaginal opening the bladder and the ureter will follow. Therefore, if incision is high on the cervix bladder or ureter can get incorporated in the incision. Here the obstruction is mostly due to ureteral kinking rather than ligation.

Precaution

Small bites of paracervical and parametrial tissue should be taken while clamping the uterosacral and the cardinal ligament. Double clamping of the uterosacral should be avoided. Adequate vesicovaginal space should be created.[3]

Bladder Injury

The incidence of bladder injury during VH is 1.86% in cases of previous cesarean section opening of the anterior pouch is difficult. Here anterior vagina is released from the cervix and sharp dissection is done at the scar towards the uterus. The bladder is then pushed upwards. Continue to operate laterally, pouch will open automatically once you reach the level.[3]

PARAVAGINAL REPAIR FOR CYSTOCELE

The sutures are placed through the white line at the level of ischial spine then passing through vagina and pubocervical fascia. There can be laceration of the bladder in case the plain of dissection is not appropriate. There is also a risk of ureteral kinking due to close proximity of the sutures.

ABDOMINAL SACROCOLPOPEXY

There can be injury to the bladder during separation of the bladder peritoneum from the vault. Sharp dissection should be done to separate the bladder.

The right ureter is prone for injury when the presacral area is exposed to fix the mesh to the anterior longitudinal ligament on the right side. The ureter should thus be identified and retracted laterally (Fig. 1).

HIGH UTEROSACRAL LIGAMENT SUSPENSION

The most common complication of high uterosacral ligament suspension (HULS) is ureteric injury. The incidence is 10.9%. The ureter is usually found 2 to 5 cm ventral and lateral to the ischial spine. The ureter is best found by applying pressure to the pelvic sidewall with the tip of the index or middle finger and sweeping from an anterior superior to a posterior inferior position. Placing the sutures into the deep dorsal aspect of the ligament is known to reduce ureteric injury.[4]

SURGERY FOR STRESS URINARY INCONTINENCE

Most common surgery used for stress urinary incontinence (SUI) is mid-urethral sling. It can be either transobturator tape (TOT) or transvaginal tape (TVT). It is seen that overall risk of urinary tract (UT) injury is lower with TOT. Using the retropubic approach, there is an approximate 5% risk of bladder or

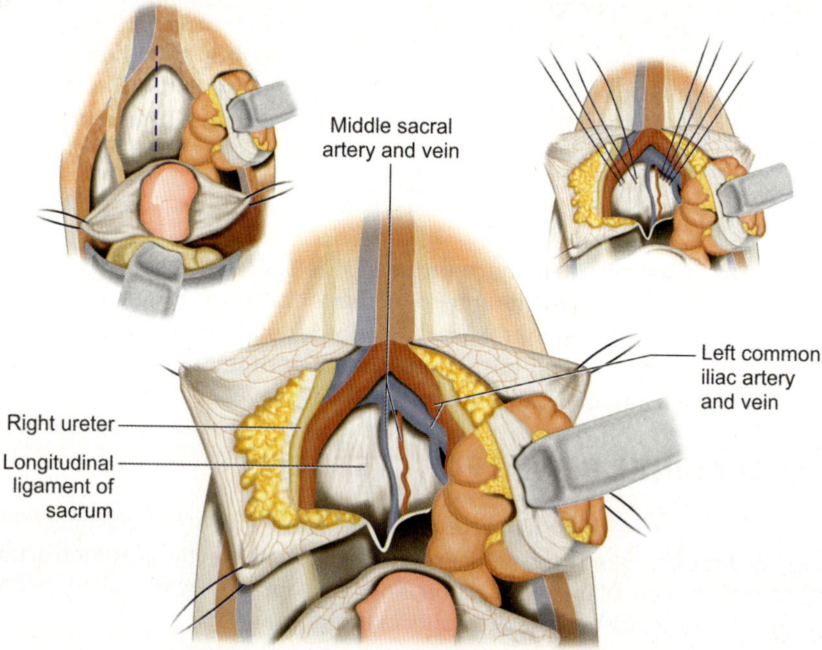

Fig. 1: Ureter in relation to anterior longitudinal ligament.

urethral perforation with trocar passage. The risk is considerably lower (<1%) with the transobturator approach.

Precaution

Expert recommendations from the American Urological Association (AUA) state that intraoperative cystoscopy should always be performed, to help minimize the risk of urinary tract injury.

Bladder Injury

In case of an inadvertent injury to bladder the trocar should be removed and replaced. Depending on the size of the injury, one might consider draining the bladder for 24 to 48 hours with an indwelling catheter. Most bladder injuries during SUI surgery are inconsequential, with no effect on outcomes.[5]

Urethral Injury

Urethral injury usually results from dissection in the wrong plane. Urethral repair should be done using 4-0 Vicryl, and the periurethral fascia should be closed. The American Urological Association's (AUA) recommendation is that *synthetic sling surgery* is contraindicated in stress incontinent patients with a concurrent urethrovaginal fistula, urethral erosion, intraoperative urethral injury and/or urethral diverticulum.[5]

SURGERY FOR MAYER-ROKITANSKY-KÜSTER-HAUSER SYNDROME (VAGINOPLASTY)

Malformation of the genital tract is often associated with anatomical variation in the urinary system like single kidney, ectopic ureter, pelvic kidney, horseshoe shape kidney, etc. Hence, it is imperative that a proper evaluation of the urinary tract should be done before posting the patient for vaginoplasty. Magnetic resonance imaging (MRI) is the gold standard for the same.

A proper preoperative idea of the anatomical variation will help us prevent inadvertent injury to the ureter or the kidney.

Bladder Injury

Creation of space for neovagina between the bladder and the rectum can cause damage to the bladder forming vesicovaginal fistula when the plane of dissection is improper. Thus, it is important that vaginal dimple be identified before placing the incision the blind vagina.

ROLE OF CYSTOURETHROSCOPY IN IDENTIFYING URINARY TRACT INJURY

An intraoperative lower urogenital tract injury is a serious problem, but an unrecognized injury is potentially disastrous and extremely dangerous and can have a drastic effect on the quality of life for the patient. It can also be a source of litigation. Complications of delayed recognition include partial or total loss of renal function, fistula formation, risks involved with additional reparative procedures, and overall poorer outcomes.

Studies have shown that use of routine intraoperative cystoscopy during major gynecologic and urogynecologic surgery might prevent sequela from lower urinary tract injuries. A study by Gilmour DT et al. showed up to 90% of unsuspected ureteral injuries and 85% of unsuspected bladder injuries were identified with the use of cystoscopy and were managed successfully intraoperatively (Fig. 2).[6]

ROLE OF PREOPERATIVE URETERIC STENTING

Prophylactic ureteric stenting is not routinely recommended. Studies have shown no significant difference in the rate of ureteric injury in patients with preoperative ureteric stenting. It has been proposed that ureteral catheters may displace the ureter into an ectopic anatomical position and may increase the likelihood of intraoperative injury.[1]

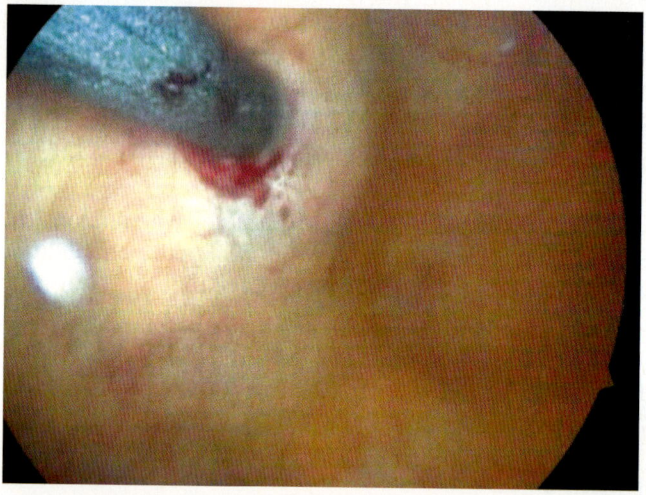

Fig. 2: Transvaginal tape (TVT) needle passed through bladder detected on cystoscopy.

INTRAOPERATIVE MANAGEMENT OF BLADDER INJURY

Bladder rent identified intraoperatively should be sutured in two or three layers with absorbable sutures 2–0 polyglactin and indwelling catheter is left in place for 2 weeks.

INTRAOPERATIVE MANAGEMENT OF URETERIC INJURY

If intraoperative ureteric injury is suspected it should be confirmed with cystoscopy and retrograde stenting. The most sensitive diagnostic study for diagnosis of a ureteral injury is a retrograde pyelogram. In case of thermal injury to the ureter retrograde stenting should be done followed by ureteric repair or reimplantation after 6 weeks. However in cases where retrograde stenting cannot be achieved a urinary diversion procedure like percutaneous nephrolithotomy is done till ureteric repair.

POSTOPERATIVE DIAGNOSIS AND MANAGEMENT OF URETERIC INJURY

Diagnosis

Early postoperative diagnosis of ureteral injury typically takes place 7 to 10 days after surgery. Symptoms include costovertebral angle tenderness, ileus, fever, and flank pain, indicating a hematoma, inflammation, or infection at the site of injury.[7] Computed tomography intravenous pyelography (CT IVP) and cystoscopy should be performed.

Management

The approach to ureteral repair depends on the cause, location, and extent of the injury. Minor trauma, such as ligature or crush injuries may be managed with stent placement and drainage of the affected area. Stents remain in place for approximately 6 weeks, followed by an intravenous pyelography (IVP) to ensure ureteral patency.[7]

Distal Ureteric Injury

As the blood supply of the distal ureteral segment may be disrupted, uretero-neocystostomy is an ideal option for distal ureteral repair. The reimplantation site should be on the posterior or anterior dome of the bladder and not on the lateral aspects. Reimplantation of the ureter on the lateral aspects of the bladder is prone to kinking with bladder filling.[1] In case of nonthermal injury, the reimplantation can be done in the same sitting intraoperatively if injury is identified. However in cases of thermal injury, reimplantation is done after 6 weeks. Postoperative diagnosis also warrants repair after 6 weeks of index surgery.

REFERENCES

1. Burks FN, Santucci RA. Management of iatrogenic ureteral injury. Ther Adv Uro. 2014;6(3): 115-24.
2. Kontogeorgos L, Vassiloppoulos P, Tentes A. Bilateral severe hydroureteronephrosis due to uterine prolapse. Br J Urol. 1985;57(3):360-1.
3. Purandare CN. Urological injuries in gynecology. J Obstet Gynecol India. 2007;57(3):203-4.
4. Post-Hysterectomy Vaginal Vault Prolapse. Green-top Guideline No.46. RCOG/BSUG Joint Guideline. 2015.
5. Nitti VW. Complications of midurethral slings and their management. Can Urol Assoc J. 2012;6(2):120-2.
6. Gilmour DT, Dwyer PL, Carey MP. Lower urinary tract injury during gynecologic surgery and its detection by intraoperative cystoscopy. Obstet Gynecol. 1999;94(2):883-9.
7. V Leanza, AF Di Prima, G Leanza, et al. How to prevent ureteral injuries during pelvic gynecological procedures. J Appl Med Sci. 2013;2(3):1-8.